WHY FAT STICKS

An Introduction To Insulin Resistance

by

Dr Guin Van Niekerk

Bloomington, IN  Milton Keynes, UK

authorHOUSE

AuthorHouse™
1663 Liberty Drive, Suite 200
Bloomington, IN 47403
www.authorhouse.com
Phone: 1-800-839-8640

AuthorHouse™ UK Ltd.
500 Avebury Boulevard
Central Milton Keynes, MK9 2BE
www.authorhouse.co.uk
Phone: 08001974150

This book is a work of non-fiction. Unless otherwise noted, the author
and the publisher make no explicit guarantees as to the accuracy of
the information contained in this book and in some cases, names of
people and places have been altered to protect their privacy.

First published by AuthorHouse 4/11/2006

ISBN: 1-4259-1539-6 (sc)

Printed in the United States of America
Bloomington, Indiana

This book is printed on acid-free paper.

I would like to dedicate this book to
my father, Louis van Niekerk.
We all miss you, Dad.

Thanks also to the Keildsons, the Kosters, the Beatties, the Drinkwaters, Michelle Roy, Debbie Cameron, Charmane Nel, Nick van Niekerk and Lesa Roderick without whom this book would never have been written. And special thanks to Christina Koster for her drawings and artistic direction.

C O N T E N T S

WHY FAT STICKS

Why *does* fat stick? This may well be one of the all – time great questions, along with " Where does love go?" and " What makes people happy?"

There are around 300 million obese people in the world today. Around two thirds of men and one half of women are overweight. When one considers the degree to which being overweight or obese affects one's health, then it becomes clear that what we have is almost a medical emergency.

> **TWO THIRDS OF MEN ARE OVERWEIGHT.**
>
> **ONE HALF OF ALL WOMEN ARE OVERWEIGHT.**
>
> **300 MILLION PEOPLE ARE OBESE.**

But why are all these people so overweight? Poor eating habits and decreasing physical activity certainly play a role in causing weight gain. But many of these overweight people do join diet programs. And they don't lose weight.

So why does fat stick?

A few decades ago, a syndrome was described which was noted to be associated with a much higher incidence than normal of cardiovascular disease, particularly sudden deaths due to heart attacks and strokes. This syndrome was named Syndrome X, and it late became known as Metabolic Syndrome or Insulin Resistance Syndrome.

It was not only discovered that the underlying cause of Metabolic Syndrome is Insulin Resistance, but also that Insulin Resistance causes

Polycystic Ovarian Syndrome (a major cause of infertility in women) and Diabetes Mellitus, and is associated with Gout and severe weight problems.

More recently it has been established that Insulin Resistance affects at least one in four people, and that one in ten normal people, who have none of the signs associated with Metabolic Syndrome, have Insulin Resistance too.

> **INSULIN RESISTANCE AFFECTS ONE IN FOUR PEOPLE.**
>
> **IT MAKES WEIGHT GAIN EASY AND WEIGHT LOSS VERY DIFFICULT.**

Insulin Resistance may well be the major reason why fat sticks. It makes weight loss extremely difficult, and weight gain ridiculously easy.

And it may be affecting you, or someone close to you.

INTRODUCTION

There comes a time in everyone's life when you stare at someone across a crowded room and you think to yourself, "Why does he/she look like that, and I look like this?"

If you have Insulin Resistance, however, the question is more likely to be something like "Why does she look like Jennifer and I look like Roseanne?" or "Why does he look like Brad and I look like Danny?"

This is because people with Insulin Resistance tend to be overweight or even obese, with a characteristic pattern of distribution of this excess weight.

> **PEOPLE WITH INSULIN RESISTANCE HAVE A VERY TYPICAL DISTRIBUTION OF ANY EXCESS WEIGHT.**
>
> **BUT YOU DON'T HAVE TO BE OVERWEIGHT TO HAVE INSULIN RESISTANCE.**

Jackie is 47 years old, and has just returned from a visit to her GP. She confides to her friend Sue, "I just can't take this anymore. Dr Jones told me that I am obese! Obese! I know that I have always been a bit too heavy, but now he tells me I am obese!" She is devastated.

Sue shakes her head slowly, as if she can't believe what she is hearing.

Jackie and Sue are both horrified by their doctor's use of the word "obese". As would any other person be. What they don't understand, is that the word obese as used by the medical profession has none of the dreadful connotations that it carries when used by the general public.

Obese is a very specific medical term which is used when a person's Body Mass Index is more than 30.

Doctors may not be the most tactful of people, but they seldom mean to be hurtful.

Still, the word obesity carries negative connotations, and because of this, we will try to avoid using it, and where we absolutely have to use it, we beg that the reader understand that it is a medical term, and is used as such.

PEOPLE WITH INSULIN RESISTANCE TEND TO HAVE WEIGHT PROBLEMS THAT ARE SELDOM DUE ONLY TO OVEREATING.

At best, Insulin Resistance is marked by a thickening around the waist. At worst, a person with Insulin Resistance is severely overweight, with all the health risks involved, as well as a poor self image. This poor self image is often due to a sense of failure that people with Insulin Resistance feel, when every diet that they try causes them to gain even more weight. And, contrary to popular belief, this weight problem is seldom exclusively due to eating excessively.

Insulin Resistance creates a situation where weight loss is extremely difficult, and weight gain ridiculously easy.

Jackie is understandably upset by her doctor's words. She has been struggling to lose weight ever since she can remember, with very little success. Whenever she joins a conventional weight loss program, she gains weight, much to everyone else's surprise and disbelief. They cannot understand how Jackie can gain weight like this. Surely she must be cheating?

But Jackie does not cheat. If anything, she eats less than her thinner friends. Despite this, she continues to have a weight problem, and today she has been told that she has high blood pressure, and that she must lose weight or she could be facing a heart attack or even a stroke. Her grandmother had a stroke, and Jackie is well aware of the unhappiness that this could cause.

" But I can't lose weight!" she sobs. "I have tried and tried, but nothing works! I don't want to have a stroke!"

Sue pats her back in sympathy. She doesn't know what to say.

So why do some people get Insulin Resistance and others don't?

The answer to this question is not a simple one.

Genetics certainly plays a part. If your parents are big, robust people, you are unlikely to be waif-like, no matter how hard you try. If your entire family is less than five feet tall, you are not going to be chosen for that basketball team.

Similarly, if your parents have Insulin Resistance, or your family has a history of Diabetes, you will probably have Insulin Resistance, or a tendency to develop Insulin Resistance.

> ## INSULIN RESISTANCE IS OFTEN INHERITED.
>
> ## IF MEMBERS OF YOUR FAMILY HAVE TYPE 2 DIABETES OR INSULIN RESISTANCE, THERE IS A GOOD CHANCE THAT YOU WILL HAVE IT TOO.

So what is Insulin Resistance?

Insulin Resistance (IR) is a condition in which your body does not recognise or respond to the hormone insulin as it should. IR is associated with and is caused to a large degree by a specific pattern of weight distribution i.e. around the waist. This central distribution of weight is known as "central obesity" in medical terms, but we will refer to it as "central weight", because many people with insulin resistance who have this specific weight distribution, are not even overweight, let alone obese!

So this central weight causes Insulin Resistance. But you need to have a genetic predisposition first, which makes it easier for you to gain weight around the waist than it does for Jack in the corner there, who guzzles beer and fast food and stays skinny.

> **INSULIN RESISTANCE MAKES IT EASIER TO GAIN WEIGHT, ESPECIALLY AROUND THE WAIST.**
>
> **THIS "CENTRAL WEIGHT" MAKES THE INSULIN RESISTANCE WORSE.**
>
> **JUNK FOOD *MAKES* YOU FAT.**
> **INSULIN RESISTANCE *KEEPS* YOU FAT!**

It's a fairly simple equation:

$$\text{Genetic Predisposition} + \text{Lifestyle} = \text{Insulin Resistance}$$

Lifestyle tends to be a vulnerable area in today's stressful times, where making a living takes precedence over health and wellbeing, and where these are sacrificed in the name of achievement. People are too busy to prepare nutritious meals or to exercise. Instead, speed becomes ultimate, with fast food and fast cars making us fat and lazy.

But let's face it, fast foods and fast cars give us those few extra minutes to work or spend quality time with friends and family.

In a world where time is at a premium, it's not easy to look after your health.

The only problem is, once a person has Insulin Resistance, it becomes almost impossible to lose weight on conventional diets. Instead, that person tends to gain weight on these diets, which aggravates the central weight which aggravates the Insulin Resistance, so they gain even more weight.

IT'S A VICIOUS CIRCLE...
WEIGHT GAIN AGGRAVATES INSULIN RESISTANCE, WHICH AGGRAVATES WEIGHT GAIN.

FAILING TO LOSE WEIGHT, OR EVEN GAINING WEIGHT ON CONVENTIONAL DIETS IS SUGGESTIVE OF INSULIN RESISTANCE.

If they are lucky, they may stumble upon a diet that seems to work. They lose weight. They feel great. Then they go back to eating normally again and…they're back to square one!

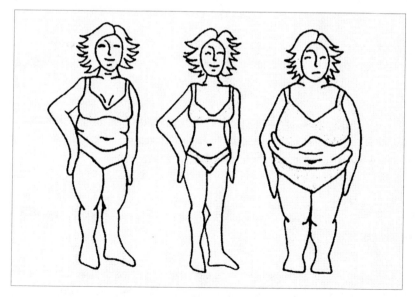

Fig 1.1 We have all seen this "Before - After - After after" scenario.

Does this pattern mean that a person definitely has Insulin Resistance?

Not necessarily.

It does, however, suggest that they *could* have Insulin Resistance.

INSULIN RESISTANCE IS SAID TO AFFECT ONE IN FOUR PEOPLE.

ONE IN TEN OTHERWISE FIT AND HEALTHY PEOPLE WILL HAVE INSULIN RESISTANCE.

Insulin Resistance is **COMMON**.

- Half of all people who have a BMI of over 30 have IR
- Half of all people with high blood pressure have IR
- One in ten people of normal weight and blood pressure have IR

BMI or Body Mass Index is a term used to describe your weight relative to your height. It is used to indicate those people at risk of developing health problems from being overweight.

A BMI of over 30 is associated with a high risk of health problems and defines the medical term "obesity". In other words, if your BMI is over 30, then your doctor may tell you that you are obese.

So... how does someone *know* when they have Insulin Resistance?

Unfortunately, in order to make a definite diagnosis of IR in a person, that person would have to undergo a specific procedure involving drips, insulin infusions, glucose infusions, and a number of blood tests. Besides being uncomfortable and time consuming, this specific test would also be expensive. As you can see, it would be impractical to test everyone in this way.

THERE IS NO SIMPLE TEST FOR THE PRESENCE OF INSULIN RESISTANCE.

So we rely on what is known in medical terms as the clinical picture. We look for a pattern, and when we see this pattern we can say, "You *may* have IR", or "You *most likely* have IR."

Once this is done, we can treat the presumptive IR, and if you feel better and lose weight, we assume that you had IR. And that you may get it again if you put on all that weight again. This is called a therapeutic trial, and is probably one of the easiest and most effective ways of pinpointing Insulin Resistance.

So when do you suspect that you have IR?

Have a look at the following checklist

- Do you or any of your family members have Type 2 Diabetes Mellitus?
- Is your body mass index more than 30?
- Is your waist: hip ratio… (see page 29)
  - More than 1.0 for men?
  - More than 0.8 for women?
- Do you have high blood pressure? (as diagnosed by your healthcare practitioner)
- Do you have high cholesterol?
- Do you have or have you had gout?

If you are a woman…

- Have you previously had Diabetes during pregnancy?
- Do you have Polycystic Ovarian Syndrome?

- Have you experienced difficulty falling pregnant?

WE LOOK FOR A SPECIFIC PATTERN IN A PERSON'S SYMPTOMS AND SIGNS, AS WELL AS THEIR FAMILY BACKGROUND.

THIS PATTERN SUGGESTS THE PRESENCE OF INSULIN RESISTANCE.

If you have ticked any of the above, you have a good chance of having IR. If you ticked more than one, your chances are quite high, and it may be a good idea to assume that you have IR.

Here is a list of additional symptoms of IR

- Cravings for sweet foods
- Weight gain on conventional high carbohydrate diets
- Otherwise unexplained tiredness
- Inappropriately increased sweating
- Moodiness or irritability or anxiety
- Rapid heart rate or palpitations
- Fluid retention; for example, swollen ankles

So there's a good chance that you have Insulin Resistance. So what?

Well besides the aesthetic problems associated with being overweight – overweight people are regarded as less than beautiful, and are discriminated against – there are many health problems.

PEOPLE WITH INSULIN RESISTANCE CRAVE SWEET FOOD, AND COMPLAIN OF CONSTANT TIREDNESS.

INSULIN RESISTANCE IS OFTEN ASSOCIATED WITH ANXIETY AND DEPRESSION.

These health problems can be categorised as :

- Mechanical problems – aching back and feet, osteoarthritis of knees, hips and back, snoring, sleep apnoea, shortness of breath.
- Cardiovascular problems – heart disease, high blood pressure.
- Metabolic problems – overweight people have increased risk of developing Diabetes, dyslipidaemias (i.e. high cholesterol) and Metabolic Syndrome (also known as Insulin Resistance Syndrome or Syndrome X)
- Cancers - of the breast in women and prostate in men
  - other cancers such as those of the oesophagus, colon and rectum, liver, gallbladder and pancreas.

BEING OVERWEIGHT OR OBESE IS ASSOCIATED WITH MANY ILLNESSES, INCLUDING SOME CANCERS.

And because central weight gain **CAUSES** Insulin Resistance (which **CAUSES** heart attacks and strokes and Diabetes) the excess central weight must be addressed.

CENTRAL WEIGHT CAUSES AND AGGRAVATES INSULIN RESISTANCE.

LOSING THE CENTRAL WEIGHT CAN IMPROVE OR EVEN CURE INSULIN RESISTANCE.

So lose weight! What's the problem? Eat less.

This is easier said than done. As mentioned previously, people with IR can't lose weight on conventional high carbohydrate diets (see chapter 2) and they feel so tired that they crave sweet foods to boost their energy levels. These sweet foods are probably the worst thing a person with Insulin Resistance can eat, because the Glycaemic Index (GI) of such foods is generally high.

Glycaemic Index is a ranking of foods based on the effect of these foods on blood glucose (also known as blood sugar).

High GI foods cause a sharp rise in blood glucose.

Low GI foods cause a slower rise in blood glucose.

HIGH GLYCAEMIC INDEX FOODS CAUSE BLOOD GLUCOSE LEVELS TO RISE RAPIDLY.

The importance of the Glycaemic index is not so much the sustained energy that low GI foods provide, but the *decrease in insulin secretion* that follows a slower release of glucose into the blood. This will be explained more fully in the next chapter, but in summary, people with Insulin Resistance cannot afford to have that insulin surge that follows a high GI meal. It prevents them from losing weight.

A RAPID RISE IN GLUCOSE MEANS A RAPID RISE IN INSULIN.

INSULIN PREVENTS FAT BREAKDOWN AND WEIGHT LOSS.

It is important to realise that it is not impossible to lose weight if you have Insulin Resistance. You need to know *what* to eat as well as how much to eat.

You need to exercise. (SORRY!)

You may even need to take medication.

But you **CAN** lose weight, and you **CAN** keep it off!

CHAPTER 1

WHAT IS INSULIN?

"A hormone is a substance secreted by certain cells in the body that exerts control over cells elsewhere in the body"

Insulin is a hormone secreted by the beta cells of the pancreas in response to a rising blood glucose level.

This situation usually occurs after a meal, when the carbohydrates (such as starches and sugars) are broken down into glucose by the digestive system. The glucose, which is the main energy source used by the body, enters the bloodstream where the rising level is detected by the pancreatic cells, which then secrete insulin.

Insulin then exerts various effects on carbohydrate, protein and fat metabolism.

CARBOHYDRATES ARE MADE UP OF SMALLER "BUILDING BLOCKS" CALLED SUGARS. GLUCOSE IS A TYPE OF SUGAR.

SUCROSE IS ALSO A SUGAR, AND CONSISTS OF GLUCOSE AND FRUCTOSE TOGETHER. SUCROSE IS THE "SUGAR" THAT WE DRINK IN TEA!

In summary:

- Insulin promotes the uptake of glucose into cells, particularly resting muscle, fat and liver cells. Nerve cells and contracting muscle cells can absorb glucose without the help of insulin!
- Insulin promotes the storage of glucose (or energy) as glycogen or fat.
- Insulin *prevents* the breakdown of glycogen and fat to form glucose.
- Insulin promotes protein formation (without insulin you don't grow)
- Insulin *prevents* protein breakdown.

> **INSULIN PROMOTES FAT AND PROTEIN FORMATION.**
>
> **INSULIN ALSO PREVENTS FAT AND PROTEIN BREAKDOWN.**

It is important to note that insulin secretion increases up to 25 times the normal level when stimulated by a high Glycaemic Index meal.

It is even more important to note that insulin levels rise in direct response to a rapid rise in blood glucose levels. The more rapid and greater the rise in blood glucose, the greater the rise in insulin secretion. *High GI foods cause more insulin to be secreted than do low GI foods.*

In other words :

HIGH GI FOODS PROMOTE FAT STORAGE AND PREVENT FAT BREAKDOWN.

This occurs in anyone, but especially in people with Insulin Resistance. This is why Glycaemic Index is so important when you are trying to lose weight.

> **HIGH GI FOODS CAUSE HIGH INSULIN LEVELS.**
>
> **HIGH GI FOODS PREVENT FAT BREAKDOWN AND THEREFORE PREVENT WEIGHT LOSS.**

Insulin secretion rises dramatically in response to a rise in blood glucose levels, which are dependent on the amount of food eaten, as well as the glycaemic index of the food.

Insulin levels remain high following a high GI meal for *a few hours.*

> **INSULIN LEVELS REMAIN HIGH FOR A FEW HOURS FOLLOWING A HIGH GLYCAEMIC INDEX MEAL.**
>
> **WITH INSULIN RESISTANCE, THESE INSULIN LEVELS CAN STAY HIGH FOR A FEW *DAYS.***

During this time   *-FAT cannot be broken down.*
                         -FAT is not used by muscle as a fuel.

Instead, fat is stored, independent of the amount of fat eaten during the meal. Carbohydrates, protein and fats are all stored as FAT.

This is clearly not an ideal situation when you are trying to lose weight (as fat, not protein).

A complete absence of glucose (or carbohydrate) is also not a good idea.

With this scenario, your insulin remains low, and this means that more fat is broken down and used as a body fuel. During this relative absence of insulin secretion, fat may be broken down, but so is protein broken down. This is because the protein sparing effect of insulin is lost. Protein forms the building blocks for most body structures, including muscle, and so a lack of insulin results in loss of muscle mass.

This can lead to a decrease in metabolic rate, because muscle uses fat as a fuel source. When you have less muscle, you burn up less fat.

A DIET WITH NO CARBOHYDRATES IN IT AT ALL RESULTS IN PROTEIN BREAKDOWN, WHICH MEANS THAT MUSCLE MASS IS LOST.

So, without any carbohydrates in your meals you would lose weight, but a large proportion of this weight would be muscle mass. You might also have bad breath and feel nauseous and tired, because the lack of insulin results in acidosis, which is due to too much fat being broken down.

This is clearly not an ideal situation either.

What we need to achieve is a situation where insulin secretion is neither too high (where fat cannot be broken down) nor too low (where protein is broken down).

This could be achieved by snacking intermittently on foods containing small amounts of carbohydrates that are more difficult to break down into glucose than sucrose (sugar) or starches. These foods would have a low carbohydrate content, as well as a low Glycaemic Index. This means that you would no longer "flood" your bloodstream with glucose. Instead, you would allow a steady trickle which gives your body the energy it needs without stimulating insulin secretion so strongly.

SOME LOW GLYCAEMIC INDEX FOODS PREVENT PROTEIN BREAKDOWN, BUT ALLOW FAT BREAKDOWN.

In a nutshell, if you avoid big meals containing lots of starch or sugar, you avoid that insulin surge, and losing weight (fat, not muscle) becomes **EASY!**

CHAPTER 2

WHAT IS INSULIN RESISTANCE?

Insulin Resistance (IR) is said to be present when the cells of your body don't respond to the hormone insulin as they should.

Insulin can be compared to a key that fits into a lock (or insulin receptor) and opens a door (through which glucose, amino acids and certain minerals pass into the cells).

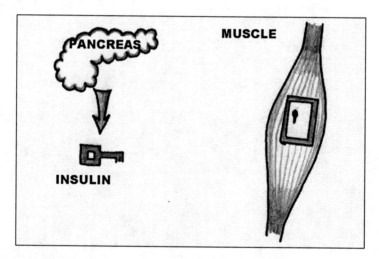

Fig 2.1

When IR occurs, the insulin is unable to activate the insulin receptor – the key does not turn the lock – and the glucose door remains closed. An overweight person with IR may have less than a quarter of the functioning insulin receptors (working locks) that a slim person has. With IR, the glucose *does* get into cells, only much slower than normal.

When IR is present, glucose can no longer be rapidly absorbed by certain tissues – resting muscle, liver and fat. Instead the glucose circulates in the blood where it is converted into fat. This fat then travels to the fatty tissues under the skin and around certain organs, where it is stored.

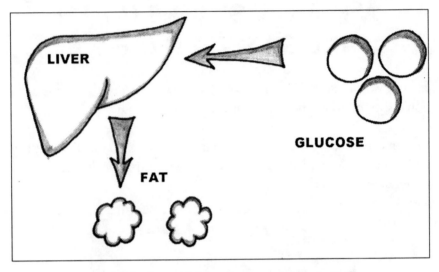

Fig 2.2 The liver converts excess glucose into fat.

NORMALLY, INSULIN CAUSES GLUCOSE TO BE TAKEN UP BY THE CELLS OF THE BODY.

WITH INSULIN RESISTANCE, GLUCOSE CIRCULATES IN THE BLOODSTREAM UNTIL IT REACHES THE LIVER, WHERE IT IS CONVERTED INTO FAT. THIS FAT IS STORED IN FATTY TISSUES THROUGHOUT THE BODY.

These fatty tissues are not only a storage space for fat; they are also metabolically active. In other words, fatty tissues (especially those around the abdomen) manufacture and secrete hormones and other substances.

These substances have been shown to aggravate Insulin Resistance.

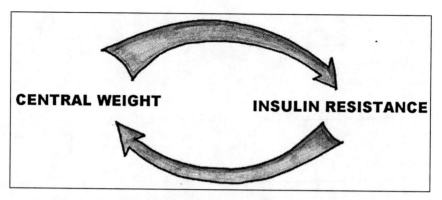

Fig 2.3 Once central weight has led to insulin resistance, a self-
perpetuating cycle begins.

**THE FAT DEPOSITED AROUND THE WAIST
IN INSULIN RESISTANT PEOPLE MAKES THE
INSULIN RESISTANCE WORSE.**

In addition to this, other effects are caused by a rising insulin level.

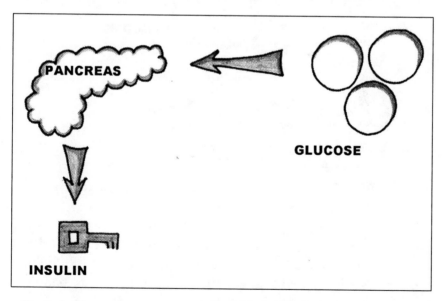

Fig 2.4 The pancreas monitors the blood glucose level and secretes
the required amount of insulin.

WITH INSULIN RESISTANCE, INSULIN LEVELS EVENTUALLY START TO RISE IN ORDER TO COMPENSATE FOR THE RESISTANCE.

THIS RISING INSULIN LEVEL CAUSES A WHOLE SET OF PROBLEMS ON ITS OWN.

THESE PROBLEMS ARE OVER AND ABOVE THE RISKS ASSOCIATED WITH OBESITY ALONE.

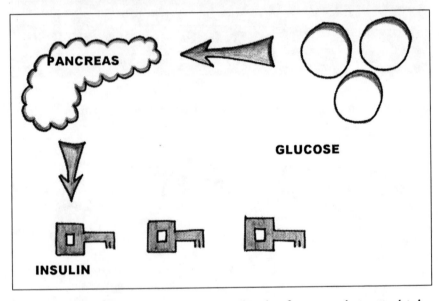

Fig 2.5 When IR occurs, the glucose levels after a meal remain high, so the pancreas secretes *more* insulin.

We believe that this hyperinsulinaemia (or raised blood insulin level) causes much of the disease process associated with Insulin Resistance, Metabolic Syndrome, and Type 2 Diabetes Mellitus; as well as conditions such as Polycystic Ovarian Syndrome.

So where do these other conditions fit in?

If we regard Insulin Resistance (IR) as a spectrum of disease, we are able to recognise the evolution of a number of clinical syndromes, including Metabolic Syndrome (MS) and Diabetes Mellitus (DM).

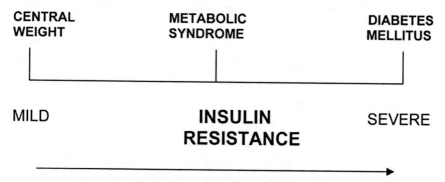

Fig 2.6 Insulin Resistance as a pathway leading to Metabolic Syndrome and Diabetes Mellitus.

Many of the other conditions associated with IR, such as Polycystic Ovarian Syndrome, Gout or skin changes, can manifest at any point along this pathway.

From Fig 2.6 we can see that it is possible to have Insulin Resistance without yet having Metabolic Syndrome or Type 2 Diabetes.

This is important to remember, because your healthcare practitioner may tell you that, from certain test results, you do not have Metabolic Syndrome or Diabetes. You may still have Insulin Resistance though!

> ### IT IS POSSIBLE TO HAVE INSULIN RESISTANCE WITHOUT HAVING CENTRAL WEIGHT, METABOLIC SYNDROME OR DIABETES.
>
> ### THESE CONDITIONS WILL MANIFEST AS THE INSULIN RESISTANCE BECOMES WORSE.

As mentioned above, hyperinsulinaemia has been shown to cause many of the disease processes associated with Insulin Resistance. For instance, raised insulin causes:

- Sympathetic over-activity – this leads to increased blood pressure, rapid heart rate, increased sweating, as well as nervous agitation and anxiety.
- Increased fatty acids in the blood which is associated with high cholesterol, and which causes plaque formation in blood vessels, and compromises the circulation of certain organs such as the heart and the brain.
- Polycystic Ovarian Syndrome – hyperinsulinaemia causes thickening of the layers around egg follicles, so instead of rupturing to release the egg (as would occur normally during ovulation) the follicle forms a cyst, and increased amounts of male hormones (androgens) are secreted (see Chapter 5)
- Sodium (salt) retention, which leads to water retention and subsequently an increased blood pressure

POLYCYSTIC OVARIAN SYNDROME IS CAUSED BY RAISED INSULIN LEVELS (OTHERWISE KNOWN AS HYPERINSULINAEMIA).

RAISED INSULIN LEVELS ALSO LEAD TO INCREASED ANXIETY AND AGITATION, AS WELL AS IRRITABILITY.

As you can see, Insulin Resistance causes a lot more than just difficulty in losing weight! IR is potentially very dangerous and it has been strongly associated with premature heart-attacks and strokes.

What causes IR in the first place?

In the introduction, we mentioned genetic predisposition as an underlying cause, as well as bad eating habits.

But what about stress?

Is it possible that stress could be a major factor in the development of central weight and subsequent IR?

Yes indeed.

> **ANOTHER VICIOUS CIRCLE: STRESS LEADS TO INSULIN RESISTANCE, WHICH LEADS TO MORE STRESS.**

Emotional and physical stress causes the secretion of the hormone cortisol by the adrenal glands. One of the most striking effects of an increased or excess cortisol production is a predominantly central distribution of fat, i.e. central weight.

This is clearly illustrated by Cushing's Syndrome, where the physical changes affecting the body are due to a *severe* excess of cortisol, which is usually either produced by a growth on the adrenal gland, or is a result of taking medication containing cortisone (and this must be taken in high doses and for a few weeks at least to cause the syndrome).

Physical features of Cushing's syndrome include:

- Increased deposition of fatty tissue around the face, the abdomen, the base if the neck and above the collarbones.
- Hirsutism and male pattern balding in women.
- Acne
- Facial redness
- Striae – which are like very large, purple stretch marks.

- Acanthosis nigricans (see page 66)

EXCESS CORTISOL, THE STRESS HORMONE, CAUSES CUSHING'S SYNDROME, WHICH IS SIMILAR TO METABOLIC SYNDROME IN SOME WAYS.

Other features of Cushing's Syndrome include

- High blood pressure
- Diabetes Mellitus
- Depression or psychosis
- Osteoporosis
- Poor wound healing

As you will see in the next chapter, there are some striking resemblances between Metabolic Syndrome and Polycystic Ovarian Syndrome, and Cushing's Syndrome.

CHAPTER 3

WHAT IS METABOLIC SYNDROME?

Metabolic Syndrome (MS) – also known as Insulin Resistance Syndrome - is a complex clinical entity, which has become extremely common as the world's population gets fatter. Some studies have shown that around 50% of people who are obese have some form of Metabolic Syndrome. When it is estimated that around 20% of the world's population is obese [i.e. having a BMI, or Body Mass Index of more than 30], this translates into about one in ten people having Metabolic Syndrome.

> **IT IS ESTIMATED THAT ONE IN TEN PEOPLE HAVE METABOLIC SYNDROME.**

The number of people affected by Insulin Resistance (IR) is probably more than this, and has been estimated by some to be around 25% of the population.

As discussed in Chapter 2, Metabolic Syndrome is a part of the Insulin Resistance spectrum of disease. It is a pre-diabetic state; in other words, it can lead to Type 2 Diabetes Mellitus (DM), but the time this takes is variable. It may be two years before the transition from MS to DM occurs, or twenty. If MS is diagnosed and treated in time, this transition may never occur.

> **METABOLIC SYNDROME OCCURS WHEN THE UNDERLYING INSULIN RESISTANCE REACHES A CERTAIN SEVERITY.**

In order to diagnose a person as having Metabolic Syndrome, your healthcare practitioner needs to have what we call a high index of suspicion. In other words, they must be alert to signs such as central weight, high blood pressure and high cholesterol, all of which may point to a diagnosis of MS.

Unfortunately, as MS has only recently been recognised as a clinical syndrome, many doctors remain unaware of the diagnostic criteria, as well as the danger of missing such a diagnosis. That is why you need to be aware if the disease, and know how a diagnosis is made. A gentle nudge in the right direction could save a life.

Current research suggests the following way of diagnosing Metabolic Syndrome: A person should have 3 out of 5 of these signs or blood test results:

1. Central Weight
2. High blood pressure
3. High triglycerides
4. Low HDL
5. High fasting blood glucose level

- the last 3 being determined by blood tests

All of these criteria will be discussed and explained in the next few pages.

YOU NEED THREE OUT OF FIVE CRITERIA IN ORDER TO BE DIAGNOSED WITH METABOLIC SYNDROME.

1. Central Weight

Central weight (known medically as central obesity – even though you may not be obese) is said to occur when your body stores fat around the organs in your abdomen, as well as in the tissue and below the skin around your waistline. This results in an increased waist : hip ratio, which remains the most reliable way of assessing central weight.

In order to calculate your waist : hip ratio you need to take two measurements –

- Waist circumference – which is said to be about halfway between the lowest part of your ribcage and the uppermost part of your hip bones.
- Hip circumference

Example 1: Bob has a waist circumference of 97cm. He measured it himself with a tape measure and remembered not to suck his stomach in! His hip circumference is 101cm

To calculate his waist : hip ratio we need to divide his waist circumference value by his hip circumference value:

$$waist{:}hip\ ratio\ =\ \frac{Waist\ circumference}{Hip\ circumference}$$

$$So\ his\ waist{:}hip\ ratio\ =\ \frac{97cm}{101cm}\ =\ 0.96$$

The accepted normal values for waist : hip ratio are:

- Adult male   - less than 1.0
- Adult female   - less than 0.8

Bob's waist : hip ratio is 0.96 which is less than 1.0. this means that Bob does not have central weight.

Example 2: Jemma has a waist circumference of 106cm, and a hip circumference of 108cm.

Her waist : hip ratio is therefore $\dfrac{106cm}{108cm}$

this works out to be 0.98.

If this value belonged to a man, he would not have central weight, but because the upper limit of normal for woman is 0.8, Jemma by definition has central weight.

> **WAIST TO HIP RATIO IS THE BEST WAY OF ASSESSING CENTRAL WEIGHT.**
>
> **CENTRAL WEIGHT IS ONE OF THE BEST PREDICTORS OF INSULIN RESISTANCE.**

Although waist : hip ratio is the best predictor of possible Metabolic Syndrome, absolute waist circumference values may also be used.

The accepted normal waist circumferences are:

- For an adult male - less than 102cm (40in)
- For an adult female - less than 88cm (35in)

> **NORMAL WAIST:HIP RATIOS ARE DIFFERENT FOR MEN AND WOMEN.**
>
> **WAIST CIRCUMFERENCE ALONE MAY ALSO BE USED TO ASSESS CENTRAL WEIGHT.**

Another important concept that requires definition here is that of obesity. We need to define this word for the sake of being complete, but would like to remind the reader that "obese" in this context is a clinical term, and should be regarded as such.

Obesity is basically a condition involving the accumulation of excess fat in the body. It can be measured objectively in a variety of ways, the most commonly used of which is the Body Mass Index (BMI).

- A normal BMI by definition lies between 18.5 and 24.9.
- Overweight is defined as having a BMI of 25 – 29.9
- Obese is defined as having a BMI of 30 or more
  (Obesity may be further divided into 3 classes:
    Class 1 obesity is a BMI of 30 – 34.9
    Class 2 obesity is a BMI of 35 – 39.9
    Class 3 obesity is a BMI of 40 or more)

The above figures can help you determine which category you fall into.

> **OBESITY INVOLVES THE ACCUMULATION OF EXCESS BODY FAT.**
>
> **OBESITY IS DEFINED AS HAVING A BODY MASS INDEX OF THIRTY OR MORE.**

To calculate your BMI:

$$BMI = \frac{weight}{height^2}$$

where weight is measured in kilograms and height is measured in metres.

Example 3: Bob weighs 85 kilograms (kgs) and his height is 175 centimetres (cms).

[Remember to convert the height from centimetres into meters, i.e. 175cm = 1.75m]

His BMI is therefore $\dfrac{85}{1{,}75^2}$ *= 27.75*

According to the above medical definitions, Bob is overweight, but not obese.

Now we need to differentiate between the two main types of weight distribution, i.e. central versus peripheral weight. In medical terms, these two patterns of weight distribution are referred to as "central obesity" and "peripheral obesity".

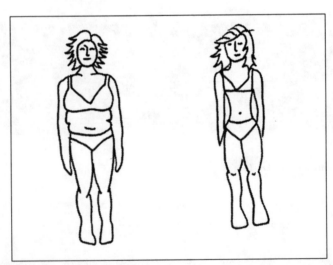

Fig 3.2 Your body shape reflects whether you have central or peripheral weight distribution. Are you an apple, or are you a pear?

A VERY IMPORTANT CONCEPT IS THE PATTERN OF DISTRIBUTION OF ANY EXCESS BODY FAT.

Central weight is the dangerous one. It is associated with heart attacks, strokes and other results of blood-vessel disease. People with central weight distribution are more likely to die suddenly, and at an earlier age than people with peripheral weight distribution. We believe that this difference is due to the nature of the fat that surrounds the waistline – it appears to be more active metabolically than fat elsewhere, and secretes hormones and other substances that cause insulin resistance, which results in hyperinsulinaemia (see Chapter 2).

CENTRAL WEIGHT DISTRIBUTION IS FAR MORE DANGEROUS THAN PERIPHERAL WEIGHT DISTRIBUTION.

Remember, central weight CAUSES Insulin Resistance, and because of this, the possibility of IR should be considered whenever some is "apple-shaped"!

2. High Blood Pressure

The second of the criteria involved in making a diagnosis of MS is high blood pressure, or hypertension. High blood pressure can be defined as an elevation of arterial blood pressure above the normal range.

BP Classification	Systolic BP	Diastolic BP
Normal	<120	<80
Pre-hypertension	120 – 139	80 – 89
Stage I hypertension	140 – 159	90 -99
Stage II hypertension	>160	>100

Table 3.1 The JNC 7 (Seventh Joint National Committee) guidelines for blood pressure levels

When your blood pressure is measured by your healthcare professional, a value will be given to you, which is usually quoted as a number over another number.

These two numbers reflect your systolic and your diastolic blood pressures.

Your systolic pressure reflects the pressure in your arteries when your heart is contracting and your diastolic pressure reflects the arterial pressure in between the contractions. Normal values for both systolic and diastolic pressures are given in Table 3.1.

In order to be diagnosed as having hypertension, you should have your blood pressure checked at least twice, with a gap of at least one week between the two measurements. Your blood pressure should be at or above 140/90 on both of these separate occasions.

YOUR BLOOD PRESSURE SHOULD BE BELOW 140/90. ANYTHING ABOVE THIS IS DEFINED AS BEING HIGH BLOOD PRESSURE.

The importance of diagnosing hypertension is well known. Prolonged elevated blood pressure has a strong association with cardiovascular disease, and consequent so-called cardiovascular events, (i.e. strokes and heart attacks). Other diseases in which hypertension has been shown to be a causative factor, are heart failure, kidney failure and dementia.

Hypertension should never be ignored, it is not "normal" to have high blood pressure as you get older!

HIGH BLOOD PRESSURE IN OLDER PEOPLE IS *NOT* "NORMAL".

The management of hypertension falls into two main categories:

1. Pharmacological – where medication is used to lower blood pressure to within normal range
2. Non-pharmacological – this category involves mainly changes in lifestyle.

> **BLOOD PRESSURE MANAGEMENT INVOLVES EITHER LIFESTYLE CHANGES ONLY, OR BOTH LIFESTYLE CHANGES AND MEDICATION.**

The pharmacological management of hypertension will be undertaken by your healthcare provider. It is, however, up to you to take the medication every day, no matter how many tablets are involved. Around 80% of hypertensives (people with high blood pressure) require more than one type of medication to control their blood pressure.

The main types of blood-pressure lowering agents are:

1. ACE inhibitors or ARB's
2. Beta blockers or alpha blockers
3. Calcium channel antagonists
4. Thiazide diuretics

An in-depth discussion of these is beyond the scope of this book. However, it is important to note that some beta blockers and thiazide diuretics have been shown to aggravate insulin resistance.

> **DO NOT STOP YOUR MEDICATION WITHOUT CONSULTING YOUR HEALTHCARE PROVIDER.**

Lifestyle changes may be as important, or even in a case of Metabolic Syndrome, more important than medication treatment of hypertension. This is especially evident in cases where hypertensive people have lost weight, sometimes as little as 5 – 10% of their mass. If we recall that central weight *causes* Insulin Resistance which *causes* (or contributes significantly to) hypertension, it is clear that sufficient weight loss weight may be curative. When compared to the alternative – ongoing treatment with costly medications, often for life – weight loss is certainly a goal that should be aimed for.

SIGNIFICANT WEIGHT LOSS AND SALT INTAKE REDUCTION ARE THE TWO MOST USEFUL LIFESTYLE CHANGES WHEN IT COMES TO LOWERING BLOOD PRESSURE.

These are the current recommended lifestyle modifications:

1. Weight loss – as mentioned above, this can *cure* Metabolic Syndrome, although having IR often makes weight loss extremely difficult. IR *prevents* you from losing weight on conventional high carbohydrate diets!

2. Salt restriction – these salty snacks must go! People with IR tend to retain sodium (salt) more readily than those without IR. This aggravates high blood pressure. Restrict salt intake to around 6 grams per day (equivalent to 2.4 grams of sodium).

3. Eat foods rich in potassium, calcium and magnesium. A list of each of these is given under the diet section of this book.

4. Stop smoking and drink moderately! A list of the recommended maximum intake for alcohol can be found in Chapter 7.

STOPPING SMOKING HELPS PREVENT MORE BLOODVESSEL DAMAGE. HIGH BLOOD PRESSURE DAMAGES BLOODVESSELS.

5. Exercise - sure you can lose weight without sweating, but exercise makes it so much easier!
   • Physical activity is a natural appetite suppressant (plus it lowers your blood pressure instead of increasing it as most other appetite suppressants do)
   • Weight training is a good way of building muscle. And muscle burns fat!

- Aerobic exercise – where you breathe faster and your heart rate rises – is great for building blood vessel bridges. Insulin resistance often means clogged arteries, and these bridges can help you get much-needed blood to areas where your circulation is already compromised.

Even more importantly, exercise does not mean you have to go to the gym. Walking, cycling, swimming, bowling and playing golf are all examples of moderate exercise. You could even wash windows vigorously or mow the lawn.

As long as you have 30 – 40 minutes of moderate exercise at least three times per week.

EXERCISE LOWERS BLOOD PRESSURE, IS A NATURAL APPETITE SUPPRESSANT, AND BUILDS MUSCLE MASS.

AND MUSCLE BURNS FAT!

6. Relax – When you have Insulin Resistance this may not be as easy as it sounds. This is because hyperinsulinaemia (raised insulin levels in the blood) causes sympathetic stimulation. This, besides causing blood-vessels to contract – and so leading to high blood pressure – can also cause emotional agitation, anxiety and an array of other symptoms such as sweating and facial flushing.

Certainly a diet that reduces your insulin levels will relieve these symptoms, but relaxation techniques such as meditation and yoga can be of value too.

PEOPLE WITH INSULIN RESISTANCE OFTEN HAVE A HIGHER STRESS LEVEL THAN OTHERS.

7. Reduce caffeine intake – Caffeine causes a degree of sympathetic stimulation too, and because of this should be avoided.

> **CAFFEINE CAN AGGRAVATE NERVOUS AGITATION, AS WELL AS RAISE BLOOD PRESSURE.**

Remember, high blood pressure (or hypertension) is a damaging, potentially fatal condition that can and MUST be treated. Hypertension does not "go away" after a course of treatment unless you lose weight and radically change your lifestyle. Don't stop your medication unless your healthcare practitioner recommends it, and even then you should check it weekly until you are one hundred percent certain that it is normal, and that it is going to stay normal.

3. High Triglycerides

Triglycerides are a type of lipid (fat) that occur in the body.

There are two basic types of lipid in the body
- **Triglycerides – or neutral fat – are the form in which fat is stored in the body, and are mainly used as an energy source. Excess carbohydrates and proteins are converted to triglycerides so that they can be stored in body fat for later use**
- **Cholesterol and phospholipids – are structural fats. They form part of the building blocks for the cell, especially structures such as the cell membrane.**

Triglycerides are derived from dietary fats, carbohydrates and proteins. They can also be mobilised from body fat stores when needed for energy.

This means that when you eat too much food your blood triglyceride levels go up. (These triglycerides are derived from your diet.) It also means that when you eat too little food your blood triglyceride levels go up! (These triglycerides are derived from your fat stores.) Other factors that can raise triglyceride levels include alcohol, oestrogen and genetic disorders.

TRIGLYCERIDES ARE EITHER DERIVED FROM YOUR DIET OR FROM YOUR BODY STORES.

Normal values for triglyceride levels may vary from country to country, but it is generally accepted that a triglyceride level over 1.7 mmol/L (or 150mg/dL) is a positive indicator of possible Metabolic Syndrome.

So why are raised triglyceride levels a problem?

Well, triglycerides are atherogenic. In other words, an increased level of triglycerides in the blood contributes to the formation of plaques which narrow blood-vessels and can lead to heart attacks and strokes.

And how does a person avoid this situation?

Ask your healthcare practitioner to do a full cholesterol profile for you. This is a blood test that should be done after an overnight fast, and it will show the levels of all the important types of cholesterol, as well as your triglyceride level.

If your triglyceride level is raised, you should avoid alcohol and only take hormone therapy under the guidance of your healthcare practitioner. Follow a healthy diet with fewer saturated fats and carbohydrates, but eat enough!

This sounds complicated. See Chapter 7 for the appropriate dietary advice.

> **RAISED TRIGLYCERIDE LEVELS CONTRIBUTE TO THE FORMATION OF PLAQUES IN BLOODVESSELS.**
>
> **THESE PLAQUES NARROW BLOODVESSELS AND CAUSE STROKES AND HEART ATTACKS.**

4. Low HDL

HDL stands for High Density Lipoprotein, which is a type of "vehicle" for cholesterol, and as such is referred to as a "type" of cholesterol. A full cholesterol profile will show the levels of HDL as well as LDL.

There are two main types of cholesterol-carrying lipoproteins – HDL and LDL. HDL contains more protein and less fat, whereas LDL contains more fat. It is believed that LDL is responsible for depositing cholesterol along arteries, and that HDL may transport cholesterol away from these arteries.

Because of this, HDL is regarded as a "good" cholesterol, and LDL a "bad" cholesterol.

HDL is a negative risk factor for atherogenic cardiovascular disease (narrowing of the arteries). In other words, a high HDL decreases your risk of heart attack or stroke. The higher it is the better.

On the other hand, a low HDL increases the risk of cardiovascular disease, and this is one of the criteria for Metabolic Syndrome.

Normal HDL levels are defined as being

- above 0.9mmol/L (40 mg/dL) for men.
- above 1.0mmol/L (50mg/dL) for women.

> **HDL IS KNOWN AS THE "GOOD" CHOLESTEROL.**
>
> **LDL IS KNOWN AS THE "BAD" CHOLESTEROL.**
>
> **A HIGH HDL LOWERS YOUR RISK OF STROKES AND HEART ATTACKS.**

Your healthcare practitioner may prescribe a cholesterol-lowering agent, or statin.

These have been shown to decrease LDL levels ("bad" cholesterol) and increase HDL levels ("good" cholesterol). They also have other effects (known as "pleiotropic effects" in medical terminology) which appear to decrease inflammation inside your blood-vessels, thereby further lowering your risk of heart attack or stroke.

> **STATINS LOWER LDL AND TRIGLYCERIDES, AND ELEVATE HDL.**

5. High fasting blood glucose level

In Chapter 2 we discussed the mechanism by which Insulin Resistance causes high blood glucose, which in turn leads to high blood insulin levels. This mechanism generally causes *prolonged* increase in blood glucose levels following a meal. In other words, your glucose levels stay high after a meal for longer than they normally should. However, with time and evolution of the disease, this prolonged increase in blood glucose level eventually persists, and your blood glucose remains high even when you have not eaten for several hours.

This results in the fifth criterion for Metabolic Syndrome: high fasting blood glucose level. High, in this case, is defined as being more than 6.1mmol/L (110mg/dL).

The blood test is done after an overnight fast. Remember not to have breakfast! Even coffee or tea is not advised, as they contain caffeine which can change your metabolism slightly and cause false results.

Management of a high fasting blood glucose level includes dietary modification (see Chapter 7), and in some cases certain medication.

The medication most likely to be used in this situation would be Metformin. Not only does Metformin lower blood glucose levels, it also targets the Insulin Resistance itself! It does this by making the insulin receptors (remember those locks?) more sensitive to insulin (the keys), and also by helping glucose get into the cell in other ways.

Metformin is a euglycaemic agent – in other words, it lowers your blood glucose if your glucose levels are high, but it does not make normal or low glucose levels even lower. So you *can't* become hypoglycaemic, or have too low a blood glucose level.

METFORMIN MAKES INSULIN RECEPTORS MORE SENSITIVE TO INSULIN, SO GLUCOSE CAN BE TAKEN UP BY THE BODY'S CELLS.

IN THIS WAY METFORMIN LOWERS BLOOD GLUCOSE AND HELPS COMBAT INSULIN RESISTANCE.

Metformin on its own causes a slight weight loss. In conjunction with a diet and exercise plan, weight loss can be significantly increased. The other effects of Insulin Resistance are also improved, and you may feel less tired and irritable as well. Your chances of developing adult onset diabetes may also be reduced by as much as 35%.

So why doesn't everyone with Insulin Resistance take Metformin?

The main reason for this is that Metformin does have side effects. These include diarrhoea, loss of appetite, nausea and a metallic taste in your mouth. It is also important to remember that Metformin may not work as well in a person who does not have a more severe degree of Insulin Resistance.

METFORMIN HAS SIDE EFFECTS AND NEEDS TO BE PRESCRIBED BY A DOCTOR.

It is best to discuss the possibility of using Metformin with your health care practitioner. Alternative medications include Pioglitazone (Actos) and Rosiglitazone (Avandia)

Once it has been established that you have three out of five of these criteria, you will be diagnosed as having Metabolic Syndrome.

The next step involves management of this condition; each criterion must be assessed and managed – blood pressure and cholesterol must be lowered with medication if necessary. Blood glucose levels should be controlled with dietary modification and medication where indicated.

However, in order to target the *cause* of IR and Metabolic Syndrome, you need to get rid of that weight around your waistline.

Remember, central weight causes IR, so get rid of the central weight and the IR will go too!

METABOLIC SYNDROME CAN BE CONTROLLED WITH MEDICATION, BUT MAY BE *CURED* BY LOSING THE EXCESS CENTRAL WEIGHT.

CHAPTER 4

DIABETES

Diabetes Mellitus, also known as Diabetes or Sugar Diabetes, is a condition which is characterised by high levels of glucose in the blood (hyperglycaemia).

There are four main types of diabetes:

1 **Type 1 Diabetes** - in which the beta cells in the pancreas are destroyed by the person's own immune system. People with Type 1 Diabetes have a deficiency in insulin.
2 **Type 2 Diabetes** - where the body tissues are resistant to insulin, so blood glucose levels rise. People with type 2 Diabetes either have high insulin levels (hyperinsulinaemia) if the pancreas is functioning well, or lower or absent insulin if the pancreas has eventually become exhausted. Ninety percent of people with Diabetes have Type 2.
3 **Other specific types of Diabetes** - these cases of high glucose can be due to many diseases, many of which cause destruction of the beta cells of the pancreas, and so lead to Diabetes. An example of this is alcoholic pancreatitis, where alcohol has toxic effects on the beta cells.
4 **Gestational Diabetes** - this is basically when a woman develops high blood glucose during pregnancy, when she has not had Diabetes before.

NINETY PERCENT OF ALL DIABETES IS DUE TO INSULIN RESISTANCE.

Diabetes, in contrast to Insulin Resistance and Metabolic Syndrome, is an easy diagnosis to make. Many people are aware of the symptoms associated with Diabetes, and the presence of high blood glucose can be confirmed with fairly simple blood test.

Here is a list of common symptoms of Diabetes to look out for:

- ☐ Thirst
- ☐ Increased urination
- ☐ Increased appetite or hunger
- ☐ Tiredness
- ☐ Blurred vision
- ☐ Weight loss

Although these symptoms may be very prominent in Type 1 Diabetes, they may not be so noticeable in Type 2 Diabetes. This is because Type 1 Diabetes tends to occur much faster than Type 2 Diabetes, which has a more gradual onset.

In order to be diagnosed as having Diabetes Mellitus, a person needs to have a blood glucose test done. If that person has fasted overnight, a blood glucose of more than 7.0 mmol/L (126 mg/dL) means that that person is Diabetic. If a person has not fasted, (i.e. the blood sample is random) a blood glucose of more than 11.1 mmol/L (200mg/dL) is diagnostic of Diabetes.

DIABETES IS DIAGNOSED WITH A SIMPLE BLOOD TEST.

ONCE DIABETES IS DIAGNOSED, BLOOD GLUCOSE LEVELS MUST BE STRICTLY MONITORED TO PREVENT COMPLICATIONS.

Other tests that may be done include a glucose tolerance test, in which you are given a fixed amount of glucose to eat, and your blood glucose levels are tested at certain intervals after this. Glycosylated haemoglobin (also known as glycated haemoglobin or HbA_{1c}) is a blood test used to monitor the control of blood glucose levels (with diet or medication) over a longer period of time – in general, it indicates a person's average blood glucose level over the previous two or three months. These results can indicate whether or not that person's blood glucose is well-controlled on the medication that they are taking. Glycosylated haemoglobin is an extremely important test once Diabetes has been diagnosed, and should be done every few months.

> **BLOOD GLUCOSE LEVELS SHOULD BE MONITORED DAILY AT HOME, AS WELL AS EVERY THREE MONTHS WITH GLYCOSYLATED HAEMOGLOBIN LEVELS.**

The reason for this is that a higher glycosylated haemoglobin result over a long period of time is associated with many of the dreaded complications of Diabetes:

- Diabetic nephropathy - raised glucose levels damage kidneys, which leads to protein in the urine as they become leaky, and eventually kidney failure.
- Diabetic retinopathy - may result in progressive loss of vision and blindness.
- Diabetic neuropathy - is where the nerves are damaged by high blood glucose levels, and may result in tingling and numbness of any area of the body, most especially the feet.
- Cardiovascular disease – involves thickening of the inner layer of blood-vessels by plaque formation. When the thickening occurs in the blood-vessels of the heart, we call it coronary artery disease, and this is what causes heart attacks. A Diabetic has the same chance of having a heart attack as does someone who as already had one!

Other complications associated with Diabetes include foot problems, which are usually as a result of both blood-vessel and nerve damage due to high blood glucose, as well as a tendency to develop infections, which is very common in diabetics.

It is important to emphasise that these complications can be largely avoided by controlling blood glucose levels properly. This control is achieved with a combination of diet, exercise, medication and regular blood sugar testing.

> **GOOD SHORT AND LONG TERM CONTROL IS VITAL TO PREVENT THE COMPLICATIONS ASSOCIATED WITH DIABETES.**

Medications used to treat Diabetes Mellitus are divided into two main groups:

1. Oral agents – which are used especially in Type 2 Diabetes. These include medications that increase insulin production by the pancreas, (eg. Glibenclamide or Gliclazide) and medications that reduce insulin resistance (i.e. Metformin,)
2. Injectable insulins – these are used mainly in Type 1 Diabetes and Gestational Diabetes, but may be necessary in Type 2 Diabetes when the pancreas has finally given up and can no longer produce insulin itself.

> **ORAL AGENTS ARE IN THE FORM OF TABLETS OR CAPSULES.**
>
> **INJECTABLE INSULINS MUST BE INJECTED UNDER THE SKIN AT LEAST ONCE DAILY.**

In most cases, Type 2 Diabetes – which is the type of Diabetes that results from Insulin Resistance, is treated with insulin sensitisers (that reduce insulin resistance) and, if necessary, insulin releasing agents (that increase insulin production by the pancreas). The fasting blood glucose levels of a person with Diabetes should be kept below 6.65mmol/L (120mg/dL). Glycosylated haemoglobin should be less than 7.0 percent.

CARE SHOULD BE TAKEN TO PREVENT THE BLOOD GLUCOSE FROM DROPPING TOO LOW (ALSO KNOWN AS HYPOGLYCAEMIA)

Type 2 Diabetes is an unpleasant illness at best and fatal at worst, but *IT CAN BE PREVENTED!* One half of all the world's diabetics have not yet been diagnosed, and by the time Diabetes is diagnosed, most of the damage has already been done. The preceding years of Insulin Resistance have resulted, in most cases, in plaque deposition in arteries, so compromising the circulation to organs such as the brain and the heart.

Having said this, a diagnosis of Diabetes need not be the life sentence it used to be. Careful management of blood glucose levels can prevent many of the associated complications.

DIABETES IS THE END RESULT OF INSULIN RESISTANCE.

IT *CAN* BE PREVENTED!

CHAPTER 5

CONDITIONS ASSOCIATED WITH INSULIN RESISTANCE

A. *POLYCYSTIC OVARIAN SYNDROME*

Pam is 27 years old. She married her childhood sweetheart about four years ago, and they have been trying to have a baby for the past three years. Pam can't understand why they have not yet succeeded...both she and her husband are young and healthy, and have never had any sexually transmitted infections. Pam does experience occasional pains in her lower abdomen, and her periods are not always regular, but she can't see how this could affect her ability to conceive.

Unfortunately, the desire to have a baby is starting to affect their relationship. Sex has become a chore, and Pam is miserable for days after every period.

Pam has seen an excellent gynaecologist, who diagnosed Polycystic Ovarian Syndrome, and gave her medication to stimulate ovulation. He also told her that she has central obesity. Pam thinks he must be mad... she has always been so careful about her weight. And those pills made her more emotional than ever.

She feels like giving up trying for a baby. But it's all she can think about.

> **POLYCYSTIC OVARIAN SYNDROME IS A COMMON CAUSE OF INFERTILITY IN WOMEN.**

Also known as the Stein-Leventhal syndrome, Polycystic Ovarian Syndrome (PCOS) is estimated to affect 6-10% of women of childbearing age.

It is believed to be the result of raised levels of insulin in the blood (hyperinsulinaemia) which causes the ovaries to secrete more male hormones (androgens) than usual. Hyperinsulinaemia also causes an imbalance in the hormones that stimulate ovulation.

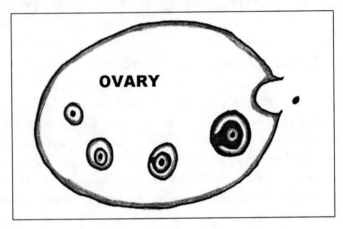

Fig 5.1 NORMAL OVARY:
Follicle maturation occurs. A follicle is a fluid-filled sac that contains one ovum (or egg). Each menstrual cycle one follicle enlarges and breaks open, releasing an egg that is transported via the Fallopian tubes to the uterus (womb).

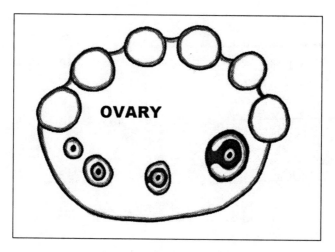

Fig 5.2 PCOS OVARY:
Complete follicle maturation fails to occur. Instead, the thickened
ovarian capsule (lining around the ovary) as well as the hormone
imbalance, results in the follicle remaining closed inside the ovary.
The egg inside the follicle is not released, so ovulation does not take
place. The follicle forms a cyst with every cycle, so the ovaries become
polycystic (meaning having many fluid-filled sacs).

**INSULIN RESISTANCE CAUSES A HORMONAL
IMBALANCE IN WOMEN, WHICH RESULTS IN
POLYCYSTIC OVARIAN SYNDROME.**

**POLYCYSTIC OVARIAN RESULTS IN FAILURE
TO OVULATE.**

The effects of excess androgens result in the classic pattern of symptoms
and signs associated with PCOS:

- Irregular or absent menstrual periods.
- Infertility.
- Increased hair growth in a male pattern of distribution – on the
  face, chest, abdomen, back, fingers and toes. This is also called
  hirsutism.

- Acne.
- Male pattern baldness – not always present.
- Pelvic pain – this pain in the lower abdomen is thought to be due to the pressure caused by cyst formation in the ovaries.

> **IRREGULAR MENSTRUATION IS ONE OF THE MORE COMMON SYMPTOMS OF POLYCYSTIC OVARIAN SYNDROME.**

Other symptoms and signs associated with PCOS are due to the underlying Insulin Resistance (IR):

- Central weight.
- High blood pressure.
- High triglyceride levels and low HDL.
- High blood glucose – this may even be high enough to be classified as Diabetes.
- Skin changes such as skin tags – these are discussed later in this chapter.

PCOS is a complex condition, and, like IR itself, is not easy to diagnose.

The name Polycystic Ovarian Syndrome is actually misleading. About 50% of women with polycystic ovaries have PCOS, and 80% of women with PCOS have polycystic ovaries. So you don't need to have polycystic ovaries in order to have PCOS.

> **POLYCYSTIC OVARIAN SYNDROME IS A *HORMONAL* DISORDER.**

Polycystic ovaries are merely one of the *signs* of the generalised hormone imbalance caused by Insulin Resistance. This hormone imbalance is known as Polycystic Ovarian Syndrome, but a better name for it might be Insulin Induced Hyperandrogenism. We will continue to refer to this syndrome as PCOS until someone does decide to change the name.

> **A WOMAN WITH PCOS DOES NOT ALWAYS HAVE CYSTS ON HER OVARIES.**
>
> **IF A WOMAN HAS OVARIES WITH CYSTS ON THEM, IT DOES NOT MEAN THAT SHE HAS PCOS.**

In order to diagnose PCOS we need to follow three steps:

Step 1 – Exclude other conditions causing a similar pattern of symptoms and signs:

- Hyperthyroidism
- Cushing's Syndrome
- Hyperprolactinaemia
- Congenial adrenal hyperplasia
- Pregnancy

Step 2 – Establish the presence of Insulin Resistance. This has been discussed in chapters 2 and 3, but basically we look for signs such as central weight, high blood pressure and cholesterol, high blood glucose. Of all these, central weight is the best predictor of IR. It may be best to assume that if central weight is present, that IR is present.

Step 3 – Establish the presence of hyperandrogenism (an excess of male hormones). Besides examination for signs such as a male pattern of hair distribution, acne, and male pattern baldness; it is also possible to do blood tests to determine levels of androgens (male hormones). These include testosterone and DHEAS. Luteinising hormone (LH) is a normally occurring female hormone, and is usually high in PCOS. This is a reflection of the generalised hormonal imbalance present.

An ultrasound or MRI scan may be done to establish the presence of cysts in the ovaries.

> # THE MOST IMPORTANT DECISION A WOMAN WITH PCOS MUST MAKE IS WHETHER OR NOT SHE WANTS CHILDREN.

The management of PCOS is fortunately a little easier than making the diagnosis. Only one important question needs to be answered:

"Is pregnancy desired?"

If a women's primary complaint is infertility, then everything must be done to promote ovulation, or release of an egg from an ovary.

And how do we do this?

Firstly – Diet and exercise. These have been shown to improve the hormonal imbalance which is at the root of the problem.

Remember:

CENTRAL WEIGHT *causes* IR *causes* PCOS

If the central weight can be eliminated from the equation, then the PCOS should improve markedly, and ovulation should occur naturally.

> # WEIGHT LOSS IS CENTRAL TO THE MANAGEMENT OF PCOS.

Secondly – Metformin. This medication has been discussed in Chapter 4. Metformin has been shown to improve Insulin Resistance, the second part of the equation.

Metformin alone has been shown to increase the occurrence of ovulation eight-fold. Metformin plus diet and exercise increases the occurrence of ovulation ten-fold. Fortunately Metformin appears not to cause and foetal abnormalities, so it is safe to fall pregnant on Metformin, although it should probably be stopped as the pregnancy progresses.

> **DIET, EXERCISE AND METFORMIN TOGETHER CAN INCREASE THE CHANCE OF OVULATING BY *TEN TIMES*.**

Thirdly — Specialist Intervention. Here a recognised fertility specialist may prescribe medication to induce ovulation, or may perform various procedures to encourage ovulation or conception, such as ovarian drilling surgery or IVF (in vitro fertilisation).

If pregnancy is not desired, the management is aimed at:

- Reducing insulin resistance.
- Regulating menstrual cycles.
- Managing the physical manifestations of PCOS, i.e. male pattern of hair distribution and acne.

> **IF A WOMAN DOES NOT WANT CHILDREN, THE TREATMENT OF PCOS IS AIMED AT REDUCING THE SYMPTOMS OF THE CONDITION.**

Insulin Resistance is managed with diet, exercise and Metformin. If high cholesterol or high blood pressure is present, these are treated with diet and the appropriate medication (see Chapter 4). Insulin Resistance is the cause of many other symptoms associated with PCOS, including mood swings, anxiety, and severe pelvic pain, especially around menstruation. These symptoms may all improve with the use of diet, exercise and Metformin.

Menstrual cycles may be regulated using the combined oral contraceptive pill. The COC most commonly used is Dianette, which contains, besides the hormones oestrogen and progesterone which are normally used in oral contraceptives, an antiandrogenic medication called cyproterone acetate. This counteracts the effects of male hormones and helps improve the hirsutism and acne.

Acne and hirsutism tend to respond to most of the above measures as well as medications such as:

- spironolactone (a diuretic that has antiandrogenic properties)
- cyproterone acetate, always in combination with the oral contraceptive (Dianette) as foetal abnormalities can result if a women falls pregnant while on cyproterone acetate.

INSULIN RESISTANCE SHOULD ALSO BE TREATED, AS THIS INCREASES THE RISK OF HEART DISEASE AND STROKES.

Finally, remember that PCOS is always due to Insulin Resistance. Treat the Insulin Resistance, and the PCOS will improve.

B. GOUT

Gout is a condition which results from the body's reaction to urate crystals. Uric acid (which forms urate crystals) forms these crystals once the blood level of uric acid reaches a certain point. The crystals are deposited in joints and tendons, and cause a marked inflammatory response by the body's own immune system. The end result of this is most commonly a severely painful, red joint.

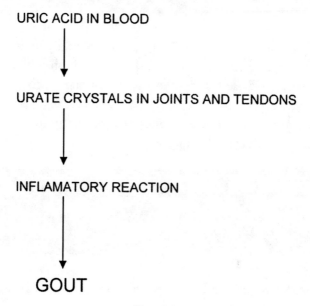

URIC ACID IN BLOOD

URATE CRYSTALS IN JOINTS AND TENDONS

INFLAMATORY REACTION

GOUT

Fig 5.3

Hyperuricaemia (raised blood uric acid levels) may also result in kidney stones. However, it is important to realise that hyperuricaemia (defined as being a uric acid level of >0,42mmol/L or 7mg/dL) does not always cause gouty arthritis or kidney stones.

GOUT OCCURS WHEN URIC ACID BUILDS UP IN THE BODY, AND URATE CRYSTALS ARE DEPOSITED IN SOFT TISSUES AND JOINTS.

THE BODY REACTS TO THESE CRYSTALS IN THE JOINTS, AND THIS RESULTS IN SEVERE PAIN AND INFLAMMATION.

Many people may have hyperuricaemia and be totally unaware of it. If this raised uric acid level is detected by chance with a blood test, the person is usually advised to decrease purine intake in the diet, and to stop medication that may be causing the raised uric acid levels. It is only when gouty arthritis or kidney stones or tophi (deposits of crystals in soft tissue) occur that medication is used to lower uric acid levels.

PURINE IS A SUBSTANCE FOUND IN MANY PROTEIN-RICH FOODS, THAT WHEN BROKEN DOWN BY THE BODY, FORMS URIC ACID.

High blood uric acid levels has many causes, which can be broadly divided into two groups:

- Increased uric acid production – this may be due to dietary factors such as high purine intake, or alcohol; as well as blood disorders such as lymphoma or polycthaemia.
- Decreased uric acid excretion by the kidneys – this may be caused by certain medications (such as thiazide diuretics) or toxins (such as alcohol). It may also be due to kidney disorders or metabolic disorders.

As you can see, alcohol gets you coming *and* going!

URIC ACID ACCUMULATES WHEN EITHER TOO MUCH IS PRODUCED, OR TOO LITTLE IS EXCRETED.

A more comprehensive list of causes of high blood uric acid levels can be found in Appendix 1.

Gout usually begins between the ages of 30 and 50 years. If it occurs earlier than this it may be due to a genetic defect in uric acid excretion by the kidney. Gout affects men far more often than women, and women who do get gout are almost always post - menopausal, and more likely to be taking medication that precipitates gout.

The most commonly affected joint in acute gout is the first metatarsophalangeal joint, which is in the large toe. Joints of the foot, ankle and knee are more commonly affected than the elbow and hand joints.

THE FIRST METATARSAL JOINT IS IN THE LARGE TOE.

So…you wake up at 2am one morning with an exquisitely painful toe that you can't even rest a bedsheet on. This is called acute gout, and is generally treated with non-steroidal anti-inflammatories (NSAID's) which settles an acute attack of gout within a few days.

Non steroidal anti-inflammatory drugs (NSAID's) should never be used by someone with a history of stomach ulcers or who is on anticoagulant therapy. Always read the enclosed leaflet of any medication being taken, and consult your healthcare practitioner if any side-effects occur.

If a large joint (i.e. the knee) is affected, a corticosteroid (cortisone) injection into the knee joint will bring quick relief.

Other methods of treatment for gout include colchicine (but the high doses used for acute gout cause *many* side effects), corticosteroids in tablet or injection form, or ACTH, (adrenocoricotropic hormone).

Once the acute attack of gout has settled, everyone breathes a sigh of relief, and hopes that it does not occur again. Fortunately there are a few measures that can be taken to help prevent another attack of gout:

- Dietary modification – foods rich in purine should be either avoided, or strictly limited. A list indicating the purine content of certain foods may be found in Appendix 2.
- AVOID ALCOHOL IN ALL FORMS! Beer is especially likely to precipitate an acute attack of gout.
- Drink at least two litres of water per day. This helps your kidneys to excrete uric acid, and prevents blood uric acid levels from rising.
- Weight loss – obesity is one of the recognised associations of gout, especially central obesity and insulin resistance!
- Occasional use of a urinary alkaliniser such as Citro-soda will increase urinary excretion of uric acid. Overuse of the alkalinisers is not recommended, as their high sodium content may elevate blood pressure.

URINARY ALKALINISERS MAY CONTAIN HIGH LEVELS OF SODIUM, AND THESE SHOULD THEREFORE BE USED SPARINGLY.

If acute gout recurs, it may be a good idea to consult your healthcare practitioner, as you may require medication to prevent ongoing deposition of urate crystals in the joints (chronic gout), as well as the recurrence of acute attacks.

Medications that may be prescribed include:

- Colchicine – this decreases the inflammatory response to urate crystals, but does not decrease blood uric acid levels. Usually given at a dosage of 0.5mg per day.
- Allopurinol – which decreases the production of uric acid, is used especially in patients with kidney failure or kidney stones.
- Probenacid and benzbromarone – these increase uric acid excretion by the kidneys. Patients on this type of medication should also take urinary alkalinisers and drink at least two litres of water per day to prevent the formation of kidney stones.

Remember, allopurinol and probenacid / benzbromarone can *cause* an acute attack of gout. To prevent this, they should be prescribed at a lower dose to start with, and in conjunction with non-steroidal anti-inflammatories or colchinine for at least 3 months.

SEVERE OR RECURRENT GOUT IS TREATED WITH MEDICATION TO LOWER URIC ACID LEVELS.

THESE MEDICATIONS SHOULD NOT BE USED DURING AN ACUTE ATTACK OF GOUT.

Gout is an unpleasant and painful condition that, in most cases, can be avoided or prevented.

Unfortunately, the concurrent existence of both gout and Insulin Resistance complicates matters, as the diet recommended in Chapter 7 is not appropriate for a gout sufferer.

MOST CASES OF GOUT CAN BE CONTROLLED BY DIETARY MEANS... AVOIDING CERTAIN PURINE-CONTAINING FOODS AND LIMITING ALCOHOL INTAKE.

Appendix 1

HYPERURICAEMIA – CAUSES

Increased uric acid production	Decreased uric acid excretion
Dietary – purine, fructose, alcohol Medications – cytotoxic drugs (drugs used in cancer), vitamin B_{12} Blood disorders – myeloma, lymphoma, leukaemia, polycythaemia Other – obesity, high triglycerides, psoriasis	Medications – diuretics (eg. thiazides, furosemide) aspirin, levodopa, TB meds (ethambutol, pyrazinamide), cyclosporin Kidney disorders – kidney failure, hypertension, polycystic kidneys. Metabolic – Type 1 Diabetes, hypothyroidism, hyperparathyroidism

Appendix 2

PURINE CONTENT OF FOODS

High...   Avoid completely:
Anchovies, bacon, codfish, haddock, kidney, liver, mussels, sardines, trout, turkey, veal, venison.

Medium...   Eat only occasionally, and in small portions:
Asparagus, beef, bouillon, chicken, crab, duck, ham, kidney beans, lentils, lima beans, lobster, mushrooms, oysters, pork, shrimp, spinach.

Low...   Unlimited amounts may be consumed:
Fizzy drinks (NOT beer!), coffee, milk, cheese and dairy products, fruits, tomatoes, green vegetables, eggs, breads, grains, pasta.

Appendix 3

MEDICATIONS TO AVOID

These medications may aggravate or precipitate gout

1 Aspirin
2 Thiazide diuretics e.g. bendrofluazide, hydrochlorothiazide
3 Other diuretics e.g. furosemide, bumetanide, torasemide
4 Levodopa e.g. co-beneldopa, co-careldopa
5 Ethambutol and Pyrazinamide
6 Cyclosporin

C. SKIN CHANGES ASSOCIATED WITH INSULIN RESISTANCE

Two of the more common skin manifestations of Insulin Resistance will be mentioned here.

1. Skin tags - These are fairly common in the normal population, but tend to occur more commonly in people with Insulin Resistance. The medical term for a skin tag is a fibroepithelial polyp, and it is completely benign (not cancer). Skin tags are usually a few millimetres in diameter, and resemble a soft, fleshy bead attached to the skin by a thin stalk of tissue. They occur especially in the groin and armpit regions, as well as around the neck; and they may be skin - coloured or darker.

    If they cause any discomfort, or if the are considered unsightly, they can be removed by your healthcare practitioner.

> **SKIN TAGS ARE ASSOCIATED WITH BUT DO NOT OCCUR EXCLUSIVELY IN INSULIN RESISTANCE.**

2. Acanthosis nigricans - This is described as a dark, velvety change that occurs in the armpit region of some people with Insulin Resistance. It does, however occur in people with adenocarcinoma), so it should be assessed by your healthcare practitioner.

CHAPTER 6

THE IMPORTANT CHAPTER

Because Insulin Resistance and its associated conditions are so complex, we would expect anyone to be a bit dazed and confused by now! Presuming, of course, that you have read the previous five chapters.

In this section we will summarise certain concepts and emphasise important points, and so hopefully leave you with an understanding of Insulin Resistance that may been lost in all the facts of the previous chapters.

Insulin is a hormone that stores energy from food eaten in times of plenty, so that this energy may be used when food is scarce. It was most likely very important for the survival of early man, who never knew where his next meal was coming from. Technology and farming, however, have changed this. Food has never been as easily available as it is today. Insulin continues to store energy derived from all this food, and the world gets fatter. Insulin also prevents the breakdown of fats, so people with high insulin levels can't lose weight, and the world *stays* fat.

> INSULIN STORES ENERGY AS FAT.
>
> THE FOOD THAT IS AVAILABLE TODAY IS VERY ENERGY DENSE.
>
> ALL THIS ENERGY IS STILL STORED VIA INSULIN, AND PEOPLE BECOME OVERWEIGHT.

Solution? Decrease insulin secretion by decreasing high GI carbohydrate (especially starch and sugar) intake. Starches and sugars are an energy source for the human body, and seldom have any other nutritional value. And if we don't use this energy by running marathons, or participating in other strenuous activities, it is stored as fat.

Insulin Resistance may be the body's way of saying, "Enough! We can't store any more energy!" Perhaps the body is trying to stop this excessive weight gain by refusing to recognise the messenger responsible for storing all this bounty.

> ## INSULIN PREVENTS THE BREAKDOWN OF FAT, AND THEREFORE PREVENTS WEIGHT LOSS.

Unfortunately, Insulin Resistance presents a whole new set of problems, including an inability to lose the weight that precipitated the Insulin Resistance in the first place!

Insulin Resistance results from a combination of these three factors:

- Genetic predisposition - a family history of Diabetes or Polycystic Ovarian Syndrome
- Lifestyle - too little exercise
  - too much of the wrong food (fast foods and ready-made meals)
- Stress - stress hormones cause weight gain around the waist-line, which heralds the onset of Insulin Resistance.

There is not much we can do about genetic predisposition, but both lifestyle and stress are areas that can be modified to prevent progression of Insulin Resistance.

Insulin Resistance should be regarded as being a spectrum of disorders

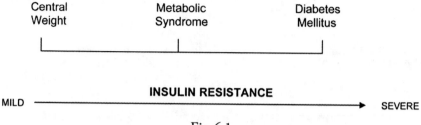

Fig 6.1

The more severe the Insulin Resistance becomes, the more likely is the development of diseases such as Metabolic Syndrome (MS) and Type 2 Diabetes Mellitus (DM). Polycystic Ovarian Syndrome (PCOS) may occur at any point along this spectrum.

As you can see from the above, it is possible for a person to have Insulin Resistance without having MS (high blood pressure, high cholesterol, high blood glucose) or DM (very high blood glucose!). Remember, PCOS is *caused* by Insulin Resistance, so if you are diagnosed as having PCOS, you definitely have Insulin Resistance.

Metabolic Syndrome – the diagnosis of MS requires 3 out of 5 of the following:

- Central weight
- High blood pressure (hypertension)
- High triglycerides
- Low HDL
- Raised fasting blood glucose

Four of the five criteria for Metabolic Syndrome are caused by hyperinsulinaemia (raised insulin levels in the blood)

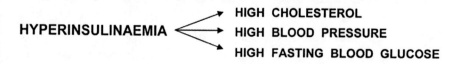

Because a diet rich in high GI carbohydrates results in hyperinsulinaemia in a person with Insulin Resistance, it can be extrapolated that high GI carbohydrates (via raised insulin levels) *cause* high cholesterol, high blood pressure and high fasting blood glucose.

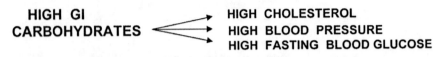

This may explain why, as was discovered in a recent study, people on a high fat, high protein diet had lower cholesterol levels after one year than people on a low fat, high carbohydrate diet. Insulin resistance may also explain why the high fat, high protein group lost substantially more weight than the low fat, high carbohydrate group.

A RECENT STUDY HAS SUGGESTED THAT HIGH CHOLESTEROL IS NOT DUE TO FATS IN THE DIET.

Maybe high blood cholesterol has very little to do with fat intake, but everything to do with carbohydrate intake! Insulin does, after all, cause the formation of triglycerides, and so increases their concentration in the blood.

So why would carbohydrates, especially those like starches and sugars, cause such a problem? The answer lies with early man, who evolved, in response to his environment, to eat animal and plant matter.

THE STARCHES AND SUGARS OF TODAY'S WORLD ARE NOT A NATURAL FOOD SOURCE !!

What caveman ever sat down to a plate of pasta, or rice, or bread or any of these starchy foods? These same foods that form the basis of our diets today, that are cheap, easily available and quick to prepare. Technology has distorted our diets, and our diets have distorted our bodies.

Cheap and easy is not always the best.

The development of Insulin Resistance has been mentioned, but once Insulin Resistance is actually present, a self-perpetuating cycle is set up:

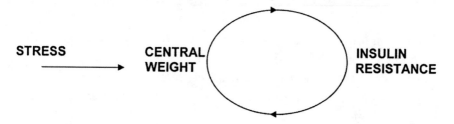

Insulin Resistance effectively prevents fat breakdown and weight loss on conventional high carbohydrate diets. In this way, central weight is perpetuated, and often made worse. A person with IR tends to just get bigger and bigger and bigger, with relief coming only in the shape of very-low-calorie and protein-only diets. Unfortunately, once "normal" eating is resumed, this happens:

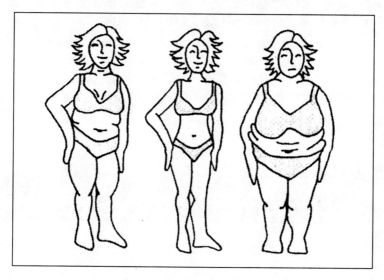

Fig 6.3

ONCE WEIGHT LOSS HAS OCCURRED ON LOW CARBOHYDRATE DIETS, PEOPLE TEND TO GO BACK TO EATING CARBS AGAIN AS PART OF A SO-CALLED "NORMAL" DIET.

THIS LEADS TO WEIGHT GAIN ALL OVER AGAIN.

The reason for this is that your body goes into "starvation mode", with very low calorie diets, and your metabolic rate drops to prevent too much weight loss. And this is why a weight loss of more than 1kg per week is regarded as being a "starvation-type", or crash diet.

To avoid the above scenario, weight loss should be gradual – around 500 grams to one kilogram per week. Once the weight is lost, and your waist : hip ratio has normalised, then your total calorie intake may be increased until you achieve an ideal weight that does not fluctuate.

CRASH DIETS CAUSE A DROP IN THE BODY'S METABOLIC RATE, SO IT BECOMES EASIER TO GAIN WEIGHT THE NEXT TIME AROUND.

Do not return to a "normal" diet! As mentioned previously, starch and sugars are NOT a natural food source. Rather avoid these foods completely, or all that weight will just be back – and more than ever before!

STARCHES AND SUGARS SHOULD NOT BE PART OF YOUR NORMAL DIET.

Insulin Resistance causes hyperinsulinaemia (raised insulin levels), which appears to be responsible for most of the disease processes associated with Insulin Resistance.

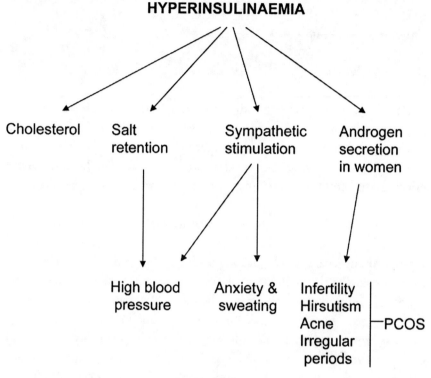

Fig 6.4

Interestingly enough, hyperinsulinaemia (raised insulin levels) causes sympathetic stimulation, which is basically the "fight / flight" response, and which involves the secretion of adrenaline and noradrenaline.

Sympathetic stimulation has a number of effects on the body – pupil dilation, increased blood pressure and heart rate, and increased mental alertness – all of which prepare the body for fighting or fleeing. Another important effect is an increase in metabolism – sometimes as much as 100%. Could it be that sympathetic stimulation in response to raised insulin levels is an attempt by the body to increase its own metabolism and so slow down that progressive deposition of energy as fat?

PEOPLE WITH INSULIN RESISTANCE AND RAISED INSULIN LEVELS TEND TO ALSO HAVE INCREASED ADRENALINE AND NORADRENALINE LEVELS, WHICH CAN MAKE THEM MORE ANXIOUS AND IRRITABLE THAN OTHERS.

Unfortunately, sympathetic stimulation results in a few fairly dangerous physical side-effects (high blood pressure, raised blood glucose and cholesterol) as well as a few less dangerous, but equally unpleasant side effects : constant tiredness, anxiety and emotional agitation. These effects have been known to improve with treatment using Metformin.

So... you suspect that you have Insulin Resistance – what to do now?

Firstly, you need to exclude (or diagnose) any dangerous conditions such as hypertension, high cholesterol, and diabetes. These will need to be managed individually by your healthcare practitioner. If you have gout, you may need to take medication to lower your uric acid levels. Also, because hyperinsulinaemia results in a tendency towards forming blood clots, or thrombosis, it may be a good idea to take ¼ aspirin (about 80mg aspirin) daily, as well as a good vitamin B supplement. Don't take aspirin if you have any sensitivity to it, or if you have previously had stomach ulcers, or if you have gout. Rather speak to your healthcare practitioner.

IF YOU SUSPECT THAT YOU HAVE INSULIN RESISTANCE, IT IS PROBABLY A GOOD IDEA TO ASSUME THAT YOU DO HAVE IT.

Secondly, the Insulin Resistance should be addressed. This may be done with dietary modification, exercise and medications, such as Metformin, which have been shown to reduce Insulin Resistance. Weight loss may eliminate central weight distribution, and lead to a natural decline in Insulin Resistance.

Thirdly, you need to avoid a recurrence or even worsening of the condition. This is vitally important, because Insulin Resistance will recur in a susceptible individual when the precipitating factors are present.

So these factors must be avoided:

- **Stress** – most people with central obesity and Insulin Resistance are able to associate the onset of weight gain and other symptoms with a particularly stressful time in their lives.

Stress causes Insulin Resistance, which in turn causes more stress (which may aggravate the Insulin Resistance)

The sympathetic stimulation response that hyperinsulinaemia causes may be largely responsible for an increased level of anxiety and sensitivity to stressful events that people with Insulin Resistance experience. It is therefore vitally important that people with Insulin Resistance are able to deal with stressful situations, so that the above "stress – IR – stress – IR" cycle can be broken.

> If you are diagnosed as having severe Depression or Anxiety, it may be necessary to have a course of anti-depressants. These should be taken for at least 6 months to a year, and should not be stopped without notifying your healthcare practitioner.

- **High Glycaemic Index carbohydrates** – especially starches and sugars, *must* be avoided indefinitely. Every time you eat a starch or sugar, your insulin levels soar, and if you have IR they stay high for a prolonged length of time. During this time you store fat, and can't break it down or lose it. Plus it leads to all the complications associated with Insulin Resistance.

YOU CAN MANAGE INSULIN RESISTANCE YOURSELF WITH MINIMAL OR NO MEDICATION.

If you have Insulin Resistance it is probably best to acknowledge that you should never eat starch or sugar again.

CHAPTER 7

INTRODUCING THE DIET

Troglodyte , *n.* a cave dweller

Insulin Resistance is a very specific problem requiring a very specific diet. Having said this, however, it is quite probable that the following eating plan (loosely referred to in this chapter as the "Troglodiet") would work for any person who wishes to lose weight. This is because the diet is specifically designed to decrease those insulin surges that generally follow a meal , and so prevent fat storage and encourage fat breakdown.

The basic premise of the Troglodiet is that the human body has not yet had time to adapt to the modern carbohydrate - rich diet that technology has given us. Instead, we believe that the eating patterns of the caveman remain the most appropriate for the human body.

Clearly it would be fairly difficult to mimic the caveman's behaviour too closely. It is probably more important to extract a few specific patterns.

> WITH INSULIN RESISTANCE, THE BEST THING TO DO IS TO EAT LIKE A CAVEMAN WOULD HAVE EATEN.

Firstly, the concept of two or three large meals per day is a relatively new one. Early man was a hunter - gatherer, which means that opportunism featured strongly in his eating behaviour. When he found food, he ate it! Food was very seldom dried and stored for later -- storage facilities would have been rudimentary at best.

So the caveman ate constantly throughout the day, munching on fresh fruit and vegetables, roots, nuts, and occasionally a handful of grain. Any animal protein would have been eaten quickly, and not as a "meat, starch and three veg combination"!

SNACK ON FRESH FOODS THROUGHOUT THE DAY.

Secondly, early man ate "organic" food, uncontaminated by pesticides, dyes, and most importantly, hormones. Who says that the hormones used to make pigs and chickens fat won't make you fat as well? In addition to this, any meat that the caveman could lay his hands on was inevitably "free - range". Not only did the caveman have to work hard to catch his meal, the meal had to work equally hard trying to get away. These energetic beasts would have been almost "fat free" as a result!

EAT ORGANIC AND FREE RANGE PRODUCTS WHERE POSSIBLE.

Thirdly, and most importantly, was the absence of certain foods in the caveman's diet. There were no starches (breads, pastas, huge floury potatoes), or sugars (sweets, chocolates, cakes) or added fats (no oils or butter to cook food in). The lack of all of these foods is most likely why no caveman ever died of a heart attack!

AVOID STARCHES, SUGARS AND ADDING OILS OR FATS TO MEALS.

The Troglodiet is a simple eating plan, with a few important guidelines that have been derived to a large degree from the eating patterns discussed above. There is only one rule that should never be bent or broken, and that is the first one.

- No starches or sugars allowed. This is really the basis for the Troglodiet.

- Avoid saturated fats, and try not to add any fats (saturated or otherwise) to your food. Bake or grill rather than fry.

- Eat intermittently throughout the day. Besides preventing hunger, this also helps to prevent those insulin surges.

- Eat a lot of food. This diet not so much about restricting calorie intake, but rather about eating the right foods. If   you eat a lot, you don't get hungry and you maintain your metabolism at its current level.

- Eat some of your protein in the morning. Protein causes a feeling of satiety, or fullness, that is stronger and lasts longer than those caused by carbohydrates and fats. If you eat protein in the morning, especially around 11am, then you should feel full for most of the day.

- Only eat when you are hungry. Although you should eat throughout the day, try to do so only when you are feeling a bit peckish. Don't eat when you are not hungry, and don't let yourself get hungry enough to want to eat everything you see!

- Drink at least 2 litres of water (or caffeine-free tea, or sugar free   colddrinks) per day. Water prevents dehydration which can   make you feel tired (and when you are tired you tend to eat to try to increase your energy levels!). Water also helps prevent uric acid levels from rising.(See Chapter 5 - Gout)

- Eat fresh organic foods. Dehydrated foods have had water removed from them, either with heat or chemicals. As such, they are processed foods. Organic foods have no pesticides or hormones that may be harming your body in as yet undetectable ways.

Please note: those suffering from kidney or liver disease, or gout, should consult their healthcare practitioners prior to using this diet plan. If you have any doubt as to your suitability, please consult your healthcare practitioner.

The quantity of food you eat should be determined by calculating your ideal body weight. This is usually expressed as a being a Body Mass Index (BMI) of between 20 and 25.

In order to calculate your ideal weight, you need to know your height.

Weight (in kgs) = BMI x Height (in metres)^2

Example 1: Bob's height is 175cm. His height in metres is 1.75m. His ideal body weight lies anywhere between a BMI of 21 to 26 (men tend to have a higher BMI range than women)

His weight should be between 21 x 1.75^2 and 26 x 1.75^2.

His ideal body weight range is from 64.3 kgs to 79.6 kgs.

For the purposes of the Troglodiet, we will assume that Bob's ideal weight is around 79 kgs. We are not trying to generate skinny people here, but healthy people.

Example 2: Jemma is 162cm tall. Her height in metres is 1.62m.

Her ideal body weight lies between a BMI of 20 and a BMI of 25.

Her weight should be between 20 x 1.62^2 and 25 x 1.62^2.

Her ideal body weight range is from 52.5 kgs to 65.6 kgs.

Realistically, Jemma should aim for a weight of about 65 kgs.

Use the following table to calculate your food intake in units:

Ideal Body Weight Range	Food Intake in Units
50 – 60 kgs	21 units
61 – 70 kgs	25 units
71 – 80 kgs	29 units
81 – 90 kgs	32 units
91 – 100 kgs	36 units

Example 1: Bob currently weighs 85 kgs. His ideal weight as calculated above is 79kgs. He is allowed 29 units of food per day on the Troglodiet.

Example 2: Jemma's ideal weight is 65 kgs. She may consume 25 units per day.

All food is divided into three broad categories in the Troglodiet: "limited", "unlimited" and "not allowed". The above unit allowance applies only to the limited foods. The unlimited foods may be eaten in unlimited quantities, and the "not allowed" foods…well, they are not allowed.

Herbs, spices and most other flavourants are permitted, also in unlimited amounts. If you have any doubts as to whether a certain condiment is allowed, read the label. If the Calorie content is less than 10 Cal per serving, then help yourself. If the energy content is not listed…avoid!

UNLIMITED FOODS

These foods have a negligible Glycaemic Index due to very low carbohydrate content, and so have a slight influence on blood glucose levels. They have many other nutrient values, however, including vitamins, minerals and fibre. They are also largely fat free.

In order to derive the maximum benefit from this diet, you should eat a number of these foods daily in fairly large portions. Any oil added to the food during preparation should be derived from the limited food unit allowance.

- Artichokes
- Asparagus
- Baby marrows / courgettes
- Brinjal
- Broccoli
- Brussels sprouts
- Butternut
- Cabbage
- Carrots
- Cauliflower
- Celery
- Chillies
- Cucumber
- Gem squash
- Green beans
- Leeks
- Lemons
- Lettuce
- Mushrooms
- Onions
- Peppers – green / red / yellow
- Pumpkin
- Radishes
- Rhubarb
- Squash
- Tomatoes

The following foods / beverages may also be consumed, although their intake should be limited to one or two portions per day.

- Artificial sweetener
- Diet sodas

- Sugar free chewing gum
- Sugar free fruit squash
- Sugar free jelly

These may be used freely when preparing food:

- Spray cooking oil
- Lemon juice
- Stock cubes *
- Soy sauce *
- Tabasco sauce
- Tomato puree
- Vinegar
- Meat extract *
- Vegetable extract *
- Salt (limit use if you have high blood pressure)*
- Pepper
- Garlic
- Ginger
- Herbs
- Spices
- Mint
- Mustard
- Parsley
- Curry powder

avoid use if suffering from high blood pressure

Unlimited beverages include:

- WATER
- Tea
- Coffee

LIMITED FOODS

These foods have either a high Glycaemic Index or a high fat percentage, or a high Calorie content.

FOOD TYPE	UNIT	VALUE
Alcohol		
• 340 ml Beer	4 units	
• 120 ml Wine		
Dry red	2 units	
Dry white	2 units	
Dry rosé	2 units	
• 25 ml Spirits		
Brandy	1 unit	
Cane	1 unit	
Gin	1 unit	
Rum	2 units	
Vodka	1 unit	
Whiskey	1 unit	
• 60 ml Sherry		
Dry	2 units	

For the purposes of the Troglodiet, fat and carbohydrate content have been defined as follows:
Fat free (FF) has less than 0.5g / 100g fat
    Low fat (LF) has a fat content less than 5g / 100g
    Medium fat (MF) has a fat content of 5 – 15g / 100g
    High fat (HF) has a fat content of more than 15g / 100g
    Very high fat (VHF) has a fat content of more than 50g / 100g
    Low carbohydrate (LC) is less than 5g / 100g
    Medium carbohydrate (MC) is 5- 20g / 100g
    High carbohydrate (HC) is more than 20g / 100g

FOOD TYPE	UNIT	VALUE
Cereals		
• Kelloggs All Bran (50g)	4 units	HC
• Swiss muesli (50g)	5 units	HC
• Raw oats (50g)	5 units	HC
Cheese		
• Camembert 100g	6 units	HF
• Cheddar 100g	8 units	HF
• Cottage cheese (low fat) 100g	2 units	LF
• Feta 100g	6 units	HF
• Gouda 100g	6 units	HF MC
Eggs		
• Boiled or raw – large	2 units	MF
• Omelette / scrambled 100g	3 units	MF
Fats / oils		
• Butter 50g	7 units	VHF
• Margarine		
Regular 50g	7 units	VHF
Floro lite 50g	3 units	VHF
• Oils		
Olive 50ml	8 units	VHF
Peanut 50ml	8 units	VHF
Soybean 50ml	8 units	VHF
Sunflower 50ml	8 units	VHF
Fish		
• Canned		
Mussels (100g)	3 units	LF
Oysters (100g)	3 units	LF
Pilchards in tomato sauce (100g)	3 units	MF
Salmon (100g)	3 units	MF
Sardines in oil (100g)	4 units	MF
Tuna in water (100g)	2 units	LF
Tuna in oil (100g)	4 units	MF

(With oil drained...always.)

FOOD TYPE	UNIT	VALUE
• Fresh fish		
Salmon (100g)	4 units	MF
Trout (100g)	3 units	LF
• Frozen fish		
Deep water hake (100g)	2 units	LF
Haddock (100g)	2 units	LF
Prawns (100g)	2 units	LF

Fruit

	UNIT	VALUE
• Apple (per 100g)	2 units	FF MC
• Avocado (100g)	4 units	MF MC
• Apricots (100g)	2 units	FF MC
• Cantaloupe (100g)	2 units	FF MC
• Cherries (100g)	2 units	FF MC
• Grapefruit (100g)	2 units	FF MC
• Kiwi fruit (100g)	4 units	FF MC
• Mango (100g)	4 units	FF MC
• Naartjies (100g)	2 units	FF MC
• Orange (100g)	2 units	FF MC
• Paw paw (100g)	4 units	FF MC
• Peach (100g)	2 units	FF MC
• Pear (100g)	2 units	FF MC
• Pineapple (100g)	4 units	FF MC
• Plums (100g)	2 units	FF MC
• Watermelon (100g)	2 units	FF MC

Meat

(All visible fat should be removed, and meat should be grilled or roasted)

	UNIT	VALUE
• Bacon – rindless back / shoulder(100g)	7 units	HF LC
• Corned beef (100g)	5 units	HF LC

FOOD TYPE	UNIT	VALUE
• Beef		
Fillet (100g)	4 units	MF
Heart (100g)	4 units	MF LC
Kidney (100g)	3 units	LF
Liver (100g)	4 units	MF LC
Lean mince (100g)	4 units	MF LC
Shoulder roast (100g)	2 units	LF
Sirloin (100g)	4 units	MF
• Biltong (100g)	5 units	MF LC
• Mutton		
Roast leg (100g)	4 units	MF
Loin chop (100g)	5 units	MF
Mince (100g)	6 units	MF
• Pork		
Roast leg (100g)	4 units	MF
Fillet (100g)	2 units	LF
• Veal roast (100g)	4 units	MF
• Venison (100g)	3 units	MF
Milk		
• Fat free (250ml)	2 units	LF MC
• Low fat (250ml)	3 units	LF MC
• Full cream (250ml)	4 units	MF MC
Nuts		
• Almonds (100g)	12 units	VHF MC
• Brazil (100g)	13 units	VHF LC
• Hazelnuts (100g)	13 units	VHF MC
• Macadamias (100g)	14 units	VHF MC
• Peanuts (100g)	12 units	HF MC
• Pecan nuts (100g)	13 units	VHF MC
• Walnuts (100g)	13 units	VHF MC

FOOD TYPE	UNIT	VALUE
Poultry		
• Chicken		
Boiled, skinless (100g)	4 units	MF
Breasts, skinless (100g)	2 units	LF
Drumsticks (100g)	4 units	MF
Thighs (100g)	4 units	MF
Livers (100g)	3 units	MF LC
• Turkey		
Roast with skin (100g)	4 units	MF
Roast without skin (100g)	3 units	LF

Protein Supplements

These may be used by vegetarians or to replace the above protein sources. Mixtures containing at least 80 – 90 % protein should be used. The unit value may be calculated by the calorie content per serving : 1 unit = 50 Calories.

Yoghurt		
• Plain low fat (250ml)	4 units	LF HC
• Plain fat free (250ml)	3 units	LF MC
• Sugar free flavoured (250ml)	3 units	LF MC

TIPS FOR EXTRA WEIGHT LOSS

1. Try to eat only the foods listed above. They have been chosen for their low carbohydrate content. For better weight loss results steer clear of the high fat foods (as far as possible).

2. Vegetarians may experience difficulty in achieving adequate protein intake. For this reason the section on "Protein supplements" was included. The taste of the products has been commented upon occasionally, and is a result of the author's opinion. These meal supplements may be used by anyone on the Troglodiet for a maximum of 15 units per day. The remaining units should consist of some of the whole foods listed above.

3. The cereal section has been included to increase fibre intake. The cereals that were selected have a low Glycaemic index, but do have a high carbohydrate content, and so should be limited to one serving (40g) per day.

4. Certain foods have been excluded, eg. banana, sausages and coconut oil. If foods are not on the list above, there is a reason for this. To use the above examples, banana has a high carbohydrate content, and so is unsuitable for someone with insulin resistance; sausages often have about 35% fat; and coconut oil contains large amounts of saturated fats which are simply bad for you!

5. If you are craving a high carbohydrate snack, try to have one before 11 am, and stick to low fat, low calorie snacks, eg. a slice of dry wholewheat toast. Limit these snacks to only once per week, and try to avoid them completely.

6. Use the weekly diet sheets on page 93. These can help you to see at a glance how many units you have eaten. Each unit is represented by a small block, with certain foods eg. fruits being limited to four units per day. Once you have eaten those units, you should shade in the appropriate blocks. You will be surprised at how much you can eat on this diet!

7. If you do not eat certain foods, eg dairy products, nuts or alcohol, transfer these units to the proteins / fats section, using the diet sheet on page 93, as shown in the example below.

Jane needs to eat 25 units per day, but she is allergic to nuts and dairy products, and does not drink alcohol. Instead, she blacks out these sections on the diet sheet and makes up the remaining units in the proteins / fats section.

WEEKLY DIET SHEET - 25 UNITS

	Alcohol	Cereals	Fruit	Milk Yoghurt	Proteins Fats *
Mon		☐☐☐☐	☐☐☐☐		☐ ☐ ☐ ☐ ☐ ☐ ☐ ☐ ☐ ☐ ☐ ☐ ☐☐

WEEKLY DIET SHEET - 36 UNITS

	Alcohol	Cereals	Fruit	Milk Yoghurt	Proteins Fats *
MON	☐☐☐☐	☐☐☐☐	☐☐☐☐	☐☐☐☐	☐☐☐☐☐ ☐☐☐☐☐ ☐☐☐☐☐ ☐☐☐☐☐
TUES	☐☐☐☐	☐☐☐☐	☐☐☐☐	☐☐☐☐	☐☐☐☐☐ ☐☐☐☐☐ ☐☐☐☐☐ ☐☐☐☐☐
WED	☐☐☐☐	☐☐☐☐	☐☐☐☐	☐☐☐☐	☐☐☐☐☐ ☐☐☐☐☐ ☐☐☐☐☐ ☐☐☐☐☐
THURS	☐☐☐☐	☐☐☐☐	☐☐☐☐	☐☐☐☐	☐☐☐☐☐ ☐☐☐☐☐ ☐☐☐☐☐ ☐☐☐☐☐
FRI	☐☐☐☐	☐☐☐☐	☐☐☐☐	☐☐☐☐	☐☐☐☐☐ ☐☐☐☐☐ ☐☐☐☐☐ ☐☐☐☐☐
SAT	☐☐☐☐	☐☐☐☐	☐☐☐☐	☐☐☐☐	☐☐☐☐☐ ☐☐☐☐☐ ☐☐☐☐☐ ☐☐☐☐☐
SUN	☐☐☐☐	☐☐☐☐	☐☐☐☐	☐☐☐☐	☐☐☐☐☐ ☐☐☐☐☐ ☐☐☐☐☐ ☐☐☐☐☐

*Proteins include meat, poultry, fish, eggs and protein supplements. Nuts may also be included in this section.

WEEKLY DIET SHEET - 32 UNITS

	Alcohol	Cereals	Fruit	Milk Yoghurt	Proteins Fats *
MON	☐☐☐☐	☐☐☐☐	☐☐☐☐	☐☐☐☐	☐☐☐☐☐ ☐☐☐☐☐ ☐☐☐☐☐ ☐
TUES	☐☐☐☐	☐☐☐☐	☐☐☐☐	☐☐☐☐	☐☐☐☐☐ ☐☐☐☐☐ ☐☐☐☐☐ ☐
WED	☐☐☐☐	☐☐☐☐	☐☐☐☐	☐☐☐☐	☐☐☐☐☐ ☐☐☐☐☐ ☐☐☐☐☐ ☐
THURS	☐☐☐☐	☐☐☐☐	☐☐☐☐	☐☐☐☐	☐☐☐☐☐ ☐☐☐☐☐ ☐☐☐☐☐ ☐
FRI	☐☐☐☐	☐☐☐☐	☐☐☐☐	☐☐☐☐	☐☐☐☐☐ ☐☐☐☐☐ ☐☐☐☐☐ ☐
SAT	☐☐☐☐	☐☐☐☐	☐☐☐☐	☐☐☐☐	☐☐☐☐☐ ☐☐☐☐☐ ☐☐☐☐☐ ☐
SUN	☐☐☐☐	☐☐☐☐	☐☐☐☐	☐☐☐☐	☐☐☐☐☐ ☐☐☐☐☐ ☐☐☐☐☐ ☐

*Proteins include meat, poultry, fish, eggs and protein supplements. Nuts may also be included in this section.

WEEKLY DIET SHEET - 29 UNITS

	Alcohol	Cereals	Fruit	Milk Yoghurt	Proteins Fats *
MON	☐☐☐☐	☐☐☐☐	☐☐☐☐	☐☐☐☐	☐☐☐☐☐ ☐☐☐☐☐ ☐☐☐
TUES	☐☐☐☐	☐☐☐☐	☐☐☐☐	☐☐☐☐	☐☐☐☐☐ ☐☐☐☐☐ ☐☐☐
WED	☐☐☐☐	☐☐☐☐	☐☐☐☐	☐☐☐☐	☐☐☐☐☐ ☐☐☐☐☐ ☐☐☐
THURS	☐☐☐☐	☐☐☐☐	☐☐☐☐	☐☐☐☐	☐☐☐☐☐ ☐☐☐☐☐ ☐☐☐
FRI	☐☐☐☐	☐☐☐☐	☐☐☐☐	☐☐☐☐	☐☐☐☐☐ ☐☐☐☐☐ ☐☐☐
SAT	☐☐☐☐	☐☐☐☐	☐☐☐☐	☐☐☐☐	☐☐☐☐☐ ☐☐☐☐☐ ☐☐☐
SUN	☐☐☐☐	☐☐☐☐	☐☐☐☐	☐☐☐☐	☐☐☐☐☐ ☐☐☐☐☐ ☐☐☐

*Proteins include meat, poultry, fish, eggs and protein supplements. Nuts may also be included in this section.

WEEKLY DIET SHEET - 25 UNITS

	Alcohol	Cereals	Fruit	Milk Yoghurt	Proteins Fats *
MON	☐☐☐☐	☐☐☐☐	☐☐☐☐	☐☐☐☐	☐☐☐ ☐☐☐ ☐☐☐
TUES	☐☐☐☐	☐☐☐☐	☐☐☐☐	☐☐☐☐	☐☐☐ ☐☐☐ ☐☐☐
WED	☐☐☐☐	☐☐☐☐	☐☐☐☐	☐☐☐☐	☐☐☐ ☐☐☐ ☐☐☐
THURS	☐☐☐☐	☐☐☐☐	☐☐☐☐	☐☐☐☐	☐☐☐ ☐☐☐ ☐☐☐
FRI	☐☐☐☐	☐☐☐☐	☐☐☐☐	☐☐☐☐	☐☐☐ ☐☐☐ ☐☐☐
SAT	☐☐☐☐	☐☐☐☐	☐☐☐☐	☐☐☐☐	☐☐☐ ☐☐☐ ☐☐☐
SUN	☐☐☐☐	☐☐☐☐	☐☐☐☐	☐☐☐☐	☐☐☐ ☐☐☐ ☐☐☐

*Proteins include meat, poultry, fish, eggs and protein supplements. Nuts may also be included in this section.

WEEKLY DIET SHEET - 21 UNITS

	Alcohol	Cereals	Fruit	Milk Yoghurt	Proteins Fats *
MON	☐☐☐☐	☐☐☐☐	☐☐☐☐	☐☐☐☐	☐☐☐☐☐
TUES	☐☐☐☐	☐☐☐☐	☐☐☐☐	☐☐☐☐	☐☐☐☐☐
WED	☐☐☐☐	☐☐☐☐	☐☐☐☐	☐☐☐☐	☐☐☐☐☐
THURS	☐☐☐☐	☐☐☐☐	☐☐☐☐	☐☐☐☐	☐☐☐☐☐
FRI	☐☐☐☐	☐☐☐☐	☐☐☐☐	☐☐☐☐	☐☐☐☐☐
SAT	☐☐☐☐	☐☐☐☐	☐☐☐☐	☐☐☐☐	☐☐☐☐☐
SUN	☐☐☐☐	☐☐☐☐	☐☐☐☐	☐☐☐☐	☐☐☐☐☐

*Proteins include meat, poultry, fish, eggs and protein supplements. Nuts may also be included in this section.

APPENDIX 1 :

GUIDELINES FOR ALCOHOL CONSUMPTION.

Men and women differ significantly in their ability to metabolise alcohol. For this reason, it is recommended that women consume less alcohol than men.

The suggested weekly limit for alcohol intake should be divided evenly throughout the week. It is not acceptable to consume the entire weekly quota in one evening, even if you have had nothing to drink in the preceding days!

The suggested weekly limit for men is 20 units per week (or three per day).

The suggested weekly limit for women is 15 units per week (or two per day).

People with diabetes or gout should try to avoid alcohol completely.

One unit of alcohol is approximately equivalent to:

- 25ml spirits
- 50ml sherry or fortified wine
- 125ml wine
- 150ml strong beer / cider
- 300ml beer / cider
- 1150ml low alcohol beer / cider

APPENDIX 2 :

FOODS HIGH IN POTASSIUM

- Apricots
- Tomato puree
- All bran
- Figs
- Dried mixed fruit
- Nuts
- Lean gammon
- Muesli
- Sardines
- Pilchards
- Veal

APPENDIX 3:

FOODS HIGH IN CALCIUM

- Milk
- Yoghurt
- Cheese
- Fish e.g. pilchards, sardines, salmon, tuna
- Vegetables e.g. broccoli, spinach, watercress, green beans
- Muesli
- Fruit e.g. apricots, figs, oranges

APPENDIX 4:

FOODS HIGH IN MAGNESIUM

- Peanuts and other types of nuts.
- Vegetables e.g. broccoli, spinach, artichoke
- Tomato puree
- Seeds e.g. pumpkin seeds
- Yoghurt
- Milk

CHAPTER 8

EXERCISE

As mentioned previously, exercise is particularly important for people with Insulin Resistance. Exercise may cause a decrease in blood pressure in the long term, as well as assisting in weight loss, which has exceptional health benefits for anyone with Insulin Resistance.

Exercise also helps you to feel fit and healthy, and takes you mind off your diet! Exercise has been shown to increase your metabolism by up to 2000% while you are exercising.

What better reason to exercise if you want to lose weight?

Current recommendations suggest that about 30 to 40 minutes of moderate exercise per day for 3 to 4 days per week is enough to boost you health and fitness significantly.

> **EXERCISE LOWERS BLOOD PRESSURE AND PROMOTES WEIGHT LOSS.**
>
> **EXERCISE IS A NATURAL APPETITE SUPPRESSANT.**
>
> **EXERCISE ALSO INCREASES YOUR METABOLIC RATE.**

The fuel type used at particular stages of exercise vary. During the first few seconds (approx 8 to 10 seconds) the phosphagen energy system is used. Here the body uses energy stored in the form of ATP and Phosphocreatine.

This system generates maximal muscle power, but can only sustain this power for a few seconds. Sprinters and weight - lifters rely almost exclusively on this system.

The second energy source used is derived from muscle glycogen, and depending on carbohydrate intake, can last up to 4 or 5 hours. The higher your carbohydrate intake, the more glycogen you store in your muscles. That is why marathon runners "carbo - load". If, however, you are not intending to run a marathon, and still wish to lose weight, it is best to avoid too many carbohydrates, so that you can make use of the third energy source available to working muscle : *fat.*

Fat is used by muscles during exercise, but the human body prefers glycogen as a fuel source, and so fat is only used extensively once muscle glycogen stores are depleted.

IF YOU EAT FEWER CARBOHYDRATES YOUR BODY BURNS FAT INSTEAD.

That is why it is important to limit your carbohydrate intake if you want to burn fat during exercise!

The amount of energy used during exercise varies greatly. It is not enough to exercise *hard* if you want to burn fat and lose weight. You need to exercise *smart.* In other words, instead of working out at a gym after you have had a high carbohydrate meal, rather hop out of bed in the morning, drink a cup of coffee (no sugar!) and go for a brisk walk. You are sure to burn more fat with the second scenario. And you can enjoy a good breakfast afterwards, too.

YOU NEED TO LEARN HOW TO EXERCISE "SMART" INSTEAD OF EXERCISING "HARD".

Moderate to strenuous exercise is more likely to cause an increased energy expenditure once exercise ceases. During exercise, even light activities burn a significant amount of energy, but once activity stops, the calorie expenditure decreases once again to where it was before. Whereas with moderate or strenuous exercise, an increase in energy consumption is maintained to a certain degree, and for up to 24 hrs afterwards.

ENERGY EXPENDITURE IS INCREASED FOR LONGER WITH MODERATE TO STRENUOUS EXERCISE.

The following tables illustrate the approximate amount of energy used by the body during each of the following activities:

Light Activity: 50 – 200 Cal / hour

Type of Activity	Energy Expenditure (Cal / hour)
Lying or sleeping	80
Sitting	100
Standing	105
Dressing	120

Moderate Activity: 200 – 350 Cal / hour

Type of Activity	Energy Expenditure (Cal / hour)
Walking at 4 km/hr	210
Cycling at 9 km/hr	240
Light intensity aerobics	240
Swimming 25 metres/min	330

Strenuous Activity: (over 350 Cal / hour)

Type of Activity	Energy Expenditure (Cal / hour)
Medium intensity aerobics	400
Walking at 7 km/hr	400
Rowing – light intensity	400
Cycling at 16 km/hr	440
Swimming 40 metres/min	480
Vigorous aerobics	600
Cycling at 21 km / hr	640
Running at 9 km/hr	640
Walking at 10 km/hr	740
Swimming 50 metres/min	790
Running at 12 km/hr	860
Running at 16 km/hr	1100

As you can see from the above figures, running fast burns more calories than most other activities, which is why running is the most popular way of exercising to lose weight.

However, if your body mass index is above 30, running may well damage certain joints, especially knee joints. For this reason we suggest the use of low impact activities such as swimming, cycling or walking. Any activity that you participate in should leave you at least slightly breathless, for example, if you go for a walk with a friend, you should have difficulty in maintaining any kind of conversation. Don't talk… walk!

ENERGY EXPENDITURE IS INCREASED FOR LONGER WITH MODERATE TO STRENUOUS EXERCISE.

And, ladies, I'm afraid it's true…women don't respond as well to exercise as men do. Women lose weight slower than most men, even if they do exercise. This may have something to do with the fact that, on average, a man's basal metabolic rate is significantly higher than a woman's. So you may have to work a lot harder than your partner to see similar results.

Exercise is unfortunately seen by many to be a tedious, time-consuming chore. This perception needs to be modified. Try buying an exercise bike and using it to work off frustration during those irritating ad breaks on television. You'll be surprised how many calories you can burn during one or two programs!

Most importantly, choose a type of exercise that you enjoy, or those good intentions may not be enough to sustain an exercise regimen!

CHAPTER 9

INSULIN RESISTANCE IN A NUTSHELL

(For those who would like an overview, this is it.)

Overeating makes you put on weight. Once your weight gain reaches a critical level, your body becomes resistant to the effects of insulin, and your insulin levels rise to try to compensate. Eventually your insulin levels stay high. This is called hyperinsulinaemia. This is more likely to occur if you have a family history of Diabetes or Insulin Resistance.

Hyperinsulinaemia has the following effects:

- It becomes impossible to lose weight. Insulin stores energy from your food as fat, and prevents fat breakdown.
- Your blood pressure rises.
- Your cholesterol levels rise.
- Your heart rate may rise, and you may experience excessive sweating, nervous agitation and anxiety.

Hyperinsulinaemia also causes the following conditions:

- Polycystic Ovarian Syndrome – a common cause of infertility in women.
- Metabolic Syndrome – also known as Insulin Resistance Syndrome, which is associated with an increased risk of heart disease and stroke.
- Diabetes – your body becomes so resistant to the high levels of insulin that your blood glucose levels eventually rise, and you become diabetic.

So when do you suspect that you may have Insulin Resistance?

Do you…

- Crave carbohydrates, especially sweet foods?
- Gain weight or lose less than expected on conventional high carbohydrate diets?
- Feel tired all the time, even though your healthcare practitioner has given you a clean bill of health?
- Sweat more than most people in similar situations?
- Feel moody or irritable or anxious for no good reasons?
- Have a rapid heart rate or get palpitations?
- Have swollen ankles that your healthcare practitioner can't find a cause for?

If you have answered yes to a few of the above questions, you may well have Insulin Resistance. So how do you know for definite?

The truth is that there is no specific test to determine whether or not you have Insulin Resistance. We have to rely on the clinical picture as a whole, with some conditions being more strongly indicative of the presence of Insulin Resistance than others.

It may be a good idea to have the following tested:

1. Your blood pressure. This should be taken at least twice, on two separate days. Use the lower of the two readings to determine if you have high blood pressure.
2. Your cholesterol levels. Two very specific levels need to be tested…your triglyceride levels and your HDL levels. This blood test should ideally be done after an overnight fast, in other words first thing in the morning after not having eaten or drunk anything from around 10pm the previous night.

Calculate your Body Mass Index:
This is calculated by dividing your weight (in kilograms) by your height (in metres) squared. See page 31.

Calculate your waist : hip ratio:

For this you will need a tape measure. See page 29.

Once you have determined the above, you can assess you risk of having Insulin Resistance using the following guidelines.

1. MAJOR FACTORS

If you have even one of these, chances are that you do have Insulin Resistance.

- Waist : hip ratio of more than
     1.0 in men
     0.8 in women
- Metabolic Syndrome (as diagnosed by your healthcare practitioner). See page 27.
- Polycystic Ovarian Syndrome (as diagnosed by your healthcare practitioner). See page 50.
- Type 2 Diabetes Mellitus (as diagnosed by your healthcare practitioner). See page 45.

2.MINOR FACTORS

Three or more of the following is highly suggestive of Insulin Resistance.

- A family history of Type 2 Diabetes.
- Body Mass Index of more than 30. See page 31.
- High blood pressure. See page 33.
- High triglycerides and low HDL. See page 39.

- Gout, currently or previously. See page 59.
- A history of diabetes during pregnancy.
- Infertility in women, or difficulty falling pregnant.

You have followed the above guidelines, and it is likely that you do have Insulin Resistance. What now?

Firstly, don't panic. Insulin resistance may not be one of the best conditions to have, but it is certainly not the worst. It is one of the few conditions that is managed to a large degree by lifestyle changes. In other words, YOU can manage this condition without the use of medication, in most cases. The only exceptions are if you have one of the following conditions, which usually require medication to prevent disastrous consequences, such as heart disease or strokes.

- High blood pressure or hypertension.
- High cholesterol (especially high triglycerides and low HDL)
- Type 2 Diabetes

Once these conditions have been either excluded or treated, the underlying Insulin Resistance can be managed by eating certain foods, and exercising, and other general measures which may help prevent the complications of Insulin Resistance. To summarise:

1. Follow a low-carbohydrate diet. See page 78.
   This will help you to lose the weight that is causing the Insulin Resistance in the first place.
2. Exercise at least three times per week.
3. Keep your salt intake down to less than 6g per day.
4. Take about 80mg of aspirin each morning. This helps to prevent heart attacks and strokes. Ask your healthcare practitioner for advice about contraindications and side effects first, though.

REMEMBER...

Carbohydrates, or carbs, aggravate Insulin Resistance by causing insulin levels to rise.

INSULIN PREVENTS FAT BREAKDOWN, SO INSULIN PREVENTS WEIGHT LOSS!

Cut out carbs and losing weight becomes easier.

GOOD LUCK!!

INSULIN RESISTANCE
CHECKLIST

1.   CENTRAL OBESITY   * optional

    [Y | N]   DATE [   ]   BMI   [   ]

                                            WAIST : HIP   [   ]
                                            RATIO

                                            WAIST   [   ]
                                            CIRCUMFERENCE

                                         * BODY FAT %   [   ]

2.   HYPERTENSION   > 140/90

    [Y | N]   DATE [   ]   Syst [   ]   Diast [   ]

                                         Syst [   ]   Diast [   ]

3.   HIGH TRIGLYCERIDES   >1.7 mmol/L

    [Y | N]   DATE [   ]   Triglyceride level [   ]

4. LOW HDL   < 0.9 mmol/L in women
                    < 1.0 mmol/L in men

    [Y | N]   DATE [   ]   HDL level [   ]

5. HIGH FASTING BLOOD GLUCOSE   > 6.1 mmol/L

    [Y | N]   DATE [   ]   Glucose level [   ]

        [GLUCOSE >7.0 mmol/L   =   DIABETIC!]

6. POLYCYSTIC OVARIAN SYNDROME

    [Y | N]   DATE [   ]   Testosterone [   ]

                                             LH [   ]

              Ultrasound done for polycystic ovaries [Y | N]

1.   GOUT/HYPERURICAEMIA

    [Y | N]   DATE [   ]   Uric acid level [   ]

GLOSSARY

Body Mass Index – a term used to describe body weight relative to height. Reflects body fat percentage, and is measured in kg/m^2.

Caffeine – a stimulant obtained from coffee and tea. Promotes wakefulness and increases mental activity.

Carbohydrate – a large group of substances including starches and sugars, from which the body derives energy. Carbohydrates are broken down to form glucose and are stored in the body as glycogen. Examples of carbohydrates include glucose, fructose, galactose, sucrose, lactose, maltose as well as starches.

Cardiovascular system – the heart and bloodvessels, also known as the circulatory system.

Cerebrovascular incident – caused by death of a section of the brain, due to interruption of the blood supply to that section. May result in paralysis of parts of the body, or speech problems or various other deficits.

Clinical – involving the study of actual patients, and the diagnosis of disease at the bedside.

Colon – the large intestine. Divided into four sections: ascending, transverse, descending and sigmoid colons.

Disaccharide – a substance consisting of two linked monosaccharide units, eg. sucrose (fructose + glucose), lactose (glucose + galactose).

Diabetes mellitus – a condition involving a relative lack of insulin, leading to an accumulation of glucose in the blood (see hyperglycaemia).

Dyslipidaemia – an abnormality of lipid concentrations in the blood.

Euglycaemic – achieving normal blood glucose levels without lowering blood glucose levels to below normal.

Gall bladder – a sac which lies below the liver, and which stores the bile that is made by the liver.

Genetics – the science of inheritance, which tries to explain how certain characteristics are passed from parents to their offspring.

Glucose – a simple sugar that is an important energy source for the body.

Heart attack – see "Myocardial infarction"

High blood pressure – see "Hypertension"

Hirsutism – increased hair growth in women in the male pattern.

Hormone – a substance produced in one part of the body which travels via the blood to another part of the body, where it acts.

Hyperglycaemia – an excess of glucose in the blood. Defined as being a blood glucose of more than 11.1 mmol/L in a random specimen.

Hypertension – increased pressure in the arteries above the normal level of 140/90 mmHg.

Hypoglycaemia – a deficiency of glucose in the blood leading to muscular weakness, incoordination, mental confusion and sweating. Defined as being a blood glucose less than 2.5 mmol/L.

Infertility – the inability to conceive in a woman, and in a man, the inability to cause conception.

Infusion – the slow injection of a substance into a vein or subcutaneous tissue.

Insulin – a hormone produced by the beta cells in the pancreas which regulates the amount of glucose in the blood.

Lipid – a group of substances including triglycerides, cholesterol and as well as other fats, steroids, phospholipids and glycolipids.

Liver – the largest gland in the body, which is situated in the upper right hand side of the abdomen.

Monosaccharide- a simple sugar eg. fructose , glucose and galactose.

Myocardial infarction – death of a segment of heart muscle, which is caused by an interruption in the blood supply to the heart. Also known as a heart attack, this may be fatal.

Obesity – a condition caused by excess fat accumulation in the body. A person is said to be obese when their BMI or Body Mass Index is more than 30.

Oesophagus – a muscular tube that extends from the throat to the stomach.

Osteoarthritis – a disease of joint cartilage which leads to pain and impaired movement in a joint.

Overweight – having a Body Mass Index of between 25 – 29.9.

Palpitations – an awareness of a persons own heartbeat. May be due to fear, exertion, or a condition causing a rapid heart rate.

Pancreas – a gland that lies behind the stomach and secretes digestive enzymes, as well as hormones such as insulin and glucagon.

Prostate – a male accessory sex gland. Enlargement may lead to difficulty passing urine.

Rectum – the section of the colon that lies between the sigmoid colon and the anus.

Sleep apnoea – a pause in breathing that can occur during sleep. Often due to obstruction of airways from relaxed muscles of the pharynx. Associated with alcohol intake and being overweight.

Starch – a substance consisting of chains of linked glucose.

Stress – a factor that threatens the health of the body or has an adverse effect on its functioning. Examples of factors causing stress include worry, injury and disease.

Stroke – see "cerebrovascular incident"

Sugar – a sweet tasting carbohydrate that dissolves in water. Includes monosaccharides and disaccharides.

Printed in the United States
89155LV00003B/291/A